EMOTION AND ATTENTION RECOGNITION BASED ON BIOLOGICAL SIGNALS AND IMAGES

Edited by **Seyyed Abed Hosseini**

Emotion and Attention Recognition Based on Biological Signals and Images
http://dx.doi.org/10.5772/62957
Edited by Seyyed Abed Hosseini

Contributors

Alberto Cruz, Belinda Le, Bir Bhanu, Manuel Vazquez-Marrufo, Xiaoming Jiang, Tiago Falk, Hussein Al Osman, Seyyed Abed Hosseini

Published by InTech

Janeza Trdine 9, 51000 Rijeka, Croatia

Publishing Process Manager Iva Simcic

Technical Editor SPi Global

Cover InTech Design team

First published February, 2017

Printed in Croatia

Additional hard copies can be obtained from orders@intechopen.com

Emotion and Attention Recognition Based on Biological Signals and Images, Edited by Seyyed Abed Hosseini

p. cm.

Print ISBN 978-953-51-2915-8

Online ISBN 978-953-51-2916-5

For EU product safety concerns:
IN TECH d.o.o., Prolaz Marije Krucifikse Kozulić 3, 51000 Rijeka, Croatia,
info@intechopen.com or visit our website at intechopen.com.

Meet the editor

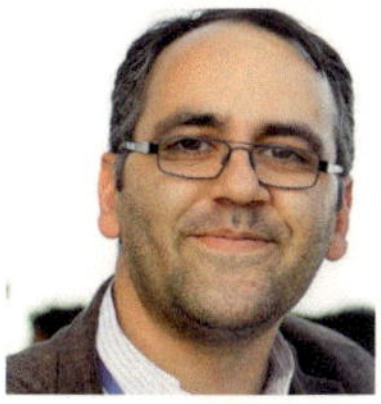

Dr. Seyyed Abed Hosseini received his BSc and MSc in Electrical Engineering and Biomedical Engineering in 2006 and 2009, respectively. He received his PhD in Electrical Engineering from the Ferdowsi University of Mashhad, Iran, in 2016. He has 10 years of teaching experience and 1 year of industry experience. He is an assistant professor at the Research Center of Biomedical Engineering, Islamic Azad University, Mashhad Branch, Iran. He has published over 50 peer-reviewed articles and book chapters in the field of emotion and attention studies. His research interests include cognitive neuroscience, biomedical signal and image processing, brain-computer interface, human-computer interaction, emotion recognition, seizure detection and prediction, neurofeedback, and human performance evaluation based on electroencephalography and event-related potential signals.

Contents

Preface

After receiving the green lights from the InTech office, the invitations went out to the senior scholars in the field from January 2016. During this 1 year of intensive efforts, all the chapters were reviewed and revised accordingly to meet high-quality standards of InTech and my vision for the whole concept of the chapters. I envision that both neuroscientists and clinical investigators will be the primary audience of this book. Moreover, the common interest of these individuals will be the application of cognitive neuroscience approaches in studies to assess or treat individuals with the related disorders based on emotion and attention.

The main focus of the book is based on emotion and attention recognition. This book is relatively brief but provides a comprehensive survey of different approaches for emotion recognition. Apart from this introductory chapter, this book has four more chapters (Chapters #2–5). The rest of this introductory chapter is given in providing brief chapters and the importance of the other proposed chapters.

Chapter 2: Multimodal Affect Recognition: Current Approaches and Challenges

This chapter provides an overview of emotion recognition, different approaches and challenges, public multimodal emotional datasets, and applications of emotion recognition. I strongly encourage the young researchers to deeply study this chapter to get a bird's-eye view of emotion and attention recognition systems.

This chapter explains that numerous studies found multimodal methods to perform as good as or better than unimodal ones. However, the improvements of multimodal systems over unimodal ones are modest when affect detection is performed on spontaneous expressions in natural settings #[15]#. Also, multimodal methods introduce new challenges that have not fully been resolved. These challenges are discussed in this chapter.

Chapter 3: Human Automotive Interaction: Affect Recognition for Motor Trend Magazine's Best Driver Car of the Year

This chapter provides two important parts of the facial emotion recognition pipeline: (1) face detection and (2) facial appearance features. This chapter proposes a face detector that unifies state-of-the-art approaches and provides quality control for face detection results, called Reference-Based Face Detection. This chapter also proposes a method for facial feature extraction that compactly encodes the spatiotemporal behavior of the face and removes the background texture, called Local Anisotropic-Inhibited Binary Patterns in Three Orthogonal Planes (LAIBP-TOP). Real-world results show promise for the automatic observation of driver inattention and stress.

Chapter 4: Affective Valence Detection from EEG Signals using Wrapper Methods

This chapter provides a valence recognition system based on a wrapper classification algorithm using EEG signals. The feature extraction in short time intervals is based on measures of the relative energies computed and certain frequency bands of the EEG signals time-locked to the stimulus presentation. These measures represent event-related desynchronization/synchronization of underlying brain neural networks. The subsequent feature selection and classification steps comprise a wrapper technique based on two different classification approaches: (1) an ensemble classifier and (2) a support vector machine classifier. The feature reduction has been used to identify the most relevant features both for intrasubject and for intersubject settings, using single-trial signals and ensemble-averaged signals, respectively. The proposed approaches allowed to identify the frontal region and beta band as the most relevant characteristics, extracted from the electrical brain activity, in order to determine the affective valence elicited by visual stimuli.

Chapter 5: Tracking the Sound of Human Affection: EEG Signals Reveal Online Decoding of Socioemotional Expression in Human Speech and Voice

This chapter provides a perspective from the latest EEG evidence on how the brain signals enlighten the neurophysiological and neurocognitive mechanisms underlying the recognition of socioemotional expression conveyed in human speech and voice, drawing upon ERP studies. Human sound can encode emotional meanings by different vocal parameters in words, real- vs. pseudospeeches, and vocalizations. Based on the ERP findings, recent development of the three-stage model in vocal processing has highlighted initial and late-stage processing of vocal emotional stimuli. These processes, depending on which ERP components they were mapped onto, can be divided into the acoustic analysis, relevance and motivational processing, fine-grained meaning analysis/integration/access, and higher-level social inference, as the unfolding of the time scale. ERP studies on vocal socioemotion, such as happiness, anger, fear, sadness, neutral, sincerity, confidence, and sarcasm in the human voice and speech, have employed different experimental paradigms such as cross-splicing, cross-modality priming, oddball, stroop, etc. Moreover, task demand and listener characteristics affect the neural responses underlying the decoding processes, revealing the role of attention deployment and interpersonal sensitivity in the neural decoding of vocal emotional stimuli. Culture affects our ability to decode emotional meaning in the voice. Neurophysiological patterns were compared between normal and abnormal emotional processing in the vocal expressions, especially schizophrenia and congenital amusia. Future directions will merit the study of human vocal expression aligning with other nonverbal cues, such as facial and body language, and the need to synchronize listener's brain potentials with other peripheral measures.

This book will provide the audiences with most recent evidences from different disciplines in brain studies on the wide range of researches in an integrative way toward *Emotion and Attention Recognition Based on Biological Signals and Images*. The hope is that the information provided in this book will trigger new researches that will help to connect basic cognitive neuroscience to clinical medicine.

Acknowledgment

Seyyed-Abed would like to thank Ms. Iva Simcic for her valuable comments and suggestions to improve the quality of this book.

Dr. Seyyed Abed Hosseini
Islamic Azad University,
Mashhad, Iran

Chapter 1

Introductory Chapter: Emotion and Attention Recognition Based on Biological Signals and Images

Seyyed Abed Hosseini

Additional information is available at the end of the chapter

http://dx.doi.org/10.5772/66483

1. Emotion and attention recognition based on biological signals and images

This chapter will attempt to introduce the different approaches for recognition of emotional and attentional states, from a historical development, focusing particularly on the recent development of the field and its specialization within psychology, cognitive neuroscience, and engineering. The basic idea of this book is to present a common framework for the neuroscientists from diverse backgrounds in the cognitive neuroscience to illustrate their theoretical and applied research findings in emotion, stress, and attention.

Biological signal processing and medical image processing have helped greatly in understanding the below-mentioned cognitive processes. Up to now, researchers and neuroscientists have studied continuously to improve the performances of the emotion and attention recognition systems (e.g., [1–10]). In spite of all of these efforts, there is still an abundance of scope for the additional researches in emotion and attention recognition based on biological signals and images. In the meantime, interpreting and modeling the notions of the brain activity, especially emotion and attention, through soft computing approaches is a challenging problem.

Emotions and attentions have an important role in our daily lives [11]. They definitely make life more challenging and interesting; however, they provide useful actions and functions that we seldom think about. Emotion and attention, due to its considerable influence on many brain activities, are important topics in the cognitive neurosciences, psychology, and biomedical engineering. These cognitive processes are core to human cognition and accessing it and being able to act have important applications ranging from basic science to applied science.

'Emotion' has many medical applications such as voice intonation, rehabilitation, autism, music therapy, and many engineering applications such as brain-computer interface (BCI), human-computer interaction (HCI), facial expression, body languages, neurofeedback, marketing, law, and robotics. In addition, 'attention' has many medical applications such as rehabilitation, autism, attention deficit disorder (ADD), attention deficit hyperactivity disorder (ADHD), attention-seeking personality disorder, and many engineering applications such as BCI, neurofeedback, decision-making, learning, and robotics.

Up to now, different definitions have been presented for the emotion and attention. According to most researchers, attention phenomenon and emotion phenomenon are not well-defined words. Kleinginna and her colleagues collected and analyzed 92 different definitions of emotion, then they made a decision that "*emotion is a complex set of interactions among subjective and objective factors, mediated by neural or hormonal systems* [12]." In addition, Solso [13] said that attention is "*the concentration of mental effort on sensory/mental events.*" In another definition, the attention function is defined as "*a cognitive brain mechanism that enables one to process relevant inputs, thoughts, or actions, whilst ignoring irrelevant or distracting ones* [14]."

In different researches, suitable techniques are usually used according to invasive or noninvasive acquisition techniques. Invasive techniques often lead to efficient systems. However, they have inherent technical difficulties such as the risks associated with surgical implantation of electrodes, stricter ethical requirements, and the fact that in humans, this can only be done in patients undergoing surgery. Therefore, noninvasive techniques such as electroencephalography (EEG), magnetoencephalography (MEG), event-related potentials (ERPs), and functional magnetic resonance imaging (fMRI) are generally preferred.

Author details

Seyyed Abed Hosseini

Address all correspondence to: hosseyni@mshdiau.ac.ir

Research Center of Biomedical Engineering, Mashhad Branch, Islamic Azad University, Mashhad, Iran

References

[1] S. Kesić and S. Z. Spasić, "Application of Higuchi's fractal dimension from basic to clinical neurophysiology: A review," *Computer Methods and Programs in Biomedicine,* vol. 133, pp. 55–70, 2016.

[2] N. Sharma and T. Gedeon, "Objective measures, sensors and computational techniques for stress recognition and classification: A survey," *Computer Methods and Programs in Biomedicine,* vol. 108, no. 3, pp. 1287–1301, 2012.

[3] S. A. Hosseini, "Classification of brain activity in emotional states using HOS analysis," *International Journal of Image, Graphics and Signal Processing*, vol. 4, no. 1, p. 21, 2012.

[4] S. A. Hosseini, and M. A. Khalilzadeh, "Emotional stress recognition system for affective computing based on bio-signals," *Journal of Biological Systems*, vol. 18, no. spec01, pp. 101–114, 2010.

[5] S. A. Hosseini, M. B. Naghibi-Sistani, and M. R. Akbarzadeh-T, "A two-dimensional brain-computer interface based on visual selective attention by Magnetoencephalograph (MEG) signals," *Tabriz Journal of Electrical Engineering*, vol. 45, no. 2, pp. 65–74, 2015.

[6] J. Chen, B. Hu, P. Moore, X. Zhang, and X. Ma, "Electroencephalogram-based emotion assessment system using ontology and data mining techniques," *Applied Soft Computing*, vol. 30, pp. 663–674, 2015.

[7] S. A. Hosseini, M. A. Khalilzadeh, M. B. Naghibi-Sistani, and V. Niazmand, "Higher order spectra analysis of EEG signals in emotional stress states," in *IEEE Second International Conference on Information Technology and Computer Science* (*ITCS*), 2010, pp. 60–63.

[8] S. A. Hosseini, M. R. Akbarzadeh-T, and M. B. Naghibi-Sistani, "Hybrid approach in recognition of visual covert selective spatial attention based on MEG signals," in *IEEE International Conference on Fuzzy Systems* (*FUZZ*), Istanbul, Turkey, 2015.

[9] S. A. Hosseini, M. R. Akbarzadeh-T, and M. B. Naghibi-Sistani, "Evaluation of visual selective attention by event related potential analysis in brain activity," *Tabriz Journal of Electrical Engineering*, vol. 45, no. 4, 2015.

[10] S. A. Hosseini, M. A. Khalilzadeh, and M. Homam, "A cognitive and computational model of brain activity during emotional stress," *Advances in Cognitive Science*, vol. 12, no. 2, pp. 1–14, 2010.

[11] C. Peter and R. Beale, *Affect and emotion in human-computer interaction: From theory to applications*, vol. 4868. Springer-Verlag Berlin Heidelberg, 2008.

[12] P. R. Kleinginna Jr and A. M. Kleinginna, "A categorized list of emotion definitions, with suggestions for a consensual definition," *Motivation and Emotion*, vol. 5, no. 4, pp. 345–379, 1981.

[13] R. L. Solso, "Cognitive Psychology," Allyn and Bacon, Pearson Education (US), 1998.

[14] M. S. Gazzaniga, R. B. Ivry, and G. R. Mangun, *Cognitive neuroscience: The biology of the mind*. Publisher: W. W. Norton & Company, 2013.

Chapter 2

Human Automotive Interaction: Affect Recognition for Motor Trend Magazine's Best Driver Car of the Year

Albert C. Cruz, Bir Bhanu and Belinda T. Le

Additional information is available at the end of the chapter

http://dx.doi.org/10.5772/65635

Abstract

Observation analysis of vehicle operators has the potential to address the growing trend of motor vehicle accidents. Methods are needed to automatically detect heavy cognitive load and distraction to warn drivers in poor psychophysiological state. Existing methods to monitor a driver have included prediction from steering behavior, smart phone warning systems, gaze detection, and electroencephalogram. We build upon these approaches by detecting cues that indicate inattention and stress from video. The system is tested and developed on data from Motor Trend Magazine's Best Driver Car of the Year 2014 and 2015. It was found that face detection and facial feature encoding posed the most difficult challenges to automatic facial emotion recognition in practice. The chapter focuses on two important parts of the facial emotion recognition pipeline: (1) face detection and (2) facial appearance features. We propose a face detector that unifies state-of-the-art approaches and provides quality control for face detection results, called reference-based face detection. We also propose a novel method for facial feature extraction that compactly encodes the spatiotemporal behavior of the face and removes background texture, called local anisotropic-inhibited binary patterns in three orthogonal planes. Real-world results show promise for the automatic observation of driver inattention and stress.

Keywords: facial emotion recognition, local appearance features, face detection

1. Introduction

In this chapter, we focus on the development of a system to track cognitive distraction and stress from facial expressions. The ultimate goal of our work is to create an early warning system to alert a driver when he/she is stressed or inattentive. This advanced facial emotion recognition technology has the potential to evolve into a human automotive interface that grants nonverbal understanding to smart cars. Motor Trend Magazine's The Enthusiast Network has collected data of a driver operating a motor vehicle on the Mazda Speedway race track for the Best Driver Car of the Year 2014 and 2015 [1]. A GoPro camera was mounted on the windshield facing the driver so that gestures and expressions could be captured naturalistically during operation of the vehicle. Attention and valence were annotated by experts according to the Fontaine/PAD model [2]. The initial goal of both tests was to detect the stress and attention of the driver as metrics for ranking cars, automatically with computer algorithms. However, affective analysis of a driver is a great challenge due to a myriad of intrinsic and extrinsic imaging conditions, extreme gaze, pose, and occlusion from gestures. In 2014, two institutions were invited to apply automatic algorithms to the task but failed. It proved too difficult to detect face region of interest (ROI) with standard algorithms [3] and it was difficult to find a facial feature-encoding scheme that gave satisfactory results. Quantification of emotion was instead carried out manually by a human expert due to these problems. In this chapter, we discuss groundbreaking findings from analysis of the Motor Trend data and share promising, novel methods for overcoming the technical challenges posed by the data.

According to the U.S. Centers for Disease Control (CDC), motor vehicle accidents (MVA) are a leading cause of injury and death in the U.S. Prevention strategies are being implemented to prevent deaths, injuries, and save medical costs. Despite this, the U.S. Department of Transportation reported that MVA increased in 2012 after 6 years of consecutive years of declining fatalities. Video-based technologies to monitor the emotion and attention of automobile drivers have the potential to curb this growing trend. Existing methods to prevent MVA include smart phone collision detection from video [4], intelligent cruise control systems [5], and gaze detection [6]. The missing link in all these prevention strategies is the holistic monitoring of the driver from video—the key participant in MVA, and the detection of cues indicating inattention and stress. The introduction of intelligent transportation systems and automotive augmented reality will exacerbate the growing problem of MVA. While one would expect autonomous/self-driving cars to decrease MVA from inattention, intelligent transportation systems will return control of the vehicle to the driver in emergency situations. This handoff can only occur safely if the vehicle operator is sufficiently attentive, though his/her attention may be elsewhere from complacency due to the auto piloting system. Augmented reality systems seek to enhance the driving experience with heads-up displays and/or head-mounted displays that can distract the vehicle operator [7]. In short, driver inattention will continue to be a significant issue with cars into the future.

2. Related work

The field of affect analysis dates back to 1872 when Charles Darwin studied the relationship between apparent expression and underlying emotional state in the book, "The Expression of the Emotions in Man and Animals [8]." Communication between humans is a complex process beyond the delivery of semantic understanding. During conversation, we communicate nonverbally with gestures, pose, and expressions. One of the first works in automatic affect analysis by computers dates to 1975 [9]. Since this seminal work, emotion recognition has found many applications in medicine [10–12], observation analysis (marketing) [13], and deception detection [14–16].

Systems to monitor the emotion and attention of vehicle operators date as far back to a 1962 patent that used steering wheel corrections as a predictor of attention and mental state [17]. Currently, there is much interest in the observation analysis of driver cognitive load, attention, and/or stress from video or biometric signals. While gaze has become a popular method for measuring attention of a driver, there is no consensus on how gaze should be monitored. Wang et al. [18] found that a driver's horizontal gaze dispersion was the most significant indicator of concentration under heavy cognitive load. Mert et al. [19] studied gaze during the handoff between manual vehicle control and autonomous piloting systems. It was found that if a driver was out of the loop it took more time to recover control of the vehicle, increasing the risk of MVA. However, a drawback to both of these methods is that it may not be possible to obtain an accurate measurement of driver gaze from video. A collaboration between AUDI AG, Volkswagen, and UC San Diego developed a video-based system for the detection of attention [20, 21]. This system focused on extracting head position and rotation using an array of cameras. We build upon state-of-the-art with an improved system that detects attention from only a single front-facing camera. In the following, we discuss the two most significant challenges to the system: face detection and facial feature encoding.

2.1. Related work in face detection

Detection of ROI is the first step of pattern recognition. In face detection, a rectangular bounding box must be computed that contains the face of an individual in the video frame. Despite significant advances to the state-of-the-art, detection of face in unconstrained facial emotion recognition scenarios is a challenging task. Occlusion, pose, and facial dynamics reduce the effectiveness of face ROI detectors. Imprecise face detection causes spurious, unrepresentative features during classification. This is a major challenge to practical applications of facial expression analysis. In Motor Trend Magazine's Best Driver Car of the Year 2014 and 2015, emotion was a metric for rating cars. In 2014, two institutions were invited to apply automatic algorithms to the task but all algorithms failed to sufficiently detect face ROI. Quantification of emotion was carried out manually by a human expert due to this problem [22].

Over the past 5 years, face detection has been carried out with the Viola and Jones algorithm (VJ) [10, 23–27]. Since the release of VJ, there have been numerous advances to face detection. Dollár et al. [28] proposed a nonrigid transformation of a model representing the face that is iteratively refined using different regressors at each iteration. Sanchez-Lozano et al. [29] proposed a novel discriminative parameterized appearance model (PAM) with an efficient regression algorithm. In discriminative PAMs, a machine- learning algorithm detects a face by fitting a model representing the object. Cootes et al. [30] proposed fitting a PAM using random forest regression voting. De Torre and Nguyen [23] proposed a novel generative PAM with a kernel-based PCA. A generative PAM models parameters such as pose and expression, whereas a discriminative PAM computes the model directly.

While the field of pattern recognition has historically been about features, ROI extraction is arguably the most important part of the entire pipeline. The adage, "garbage-in garbage-out" applies. In the AV+EC 2015 grand challenge, the Viola and Jones face detector [3] has a 6.5% detection rate and Google Picasa has a 0.07% detection rate. How does one infer the missing 93.95% of face ROIs? Among the "successfully" extracted faces, what is their quality? If one were to fill in the missing values with poor ROIs the extracted features would be erroneous and lead to a poor decision model. To address this, we propose a system that unifies current approaches and provides quality control of extraction results, called *reference-based face detection*. The method consists of two phases: (1) In training, a generic face is computed that is centered in the image. This image is used as a reference to quantify the quality of detection results in the next step. (2) In testing, multiple candidate face ROIs are detected, and the candidate ROI that best matches the reference face in the least squared sense is selected for further processing. Three different methodologies for finding the face ROIs are considered: a boosted cascade of Haar-like features, discriminative parameterized appearances, and a parts-based deformable models. These three major types of face detectors perform well in exclusive situations. Therefore, better performance can be achieved by unifying these three methods to generate multiple candidate face ROIs and quantifiably determine which candidate is the best ROI.

2.2. Related work in facial appearance features

Local binary patterns (LBP) are one of the most commonly used facial appearance features. They were originally proposed by Ojala et al. [31] as static feature descriptors that capture texture features within a single frame. LBP encode microtextures by comparing the current pixel to neighboring pixels. Differences are recorded at the bit level, e.g., if the top pixel is greater than the middle pixel a specific bit is set. Identical microtextures will take on the same integer value. There have been many improvements and variations of LBP over the years as the problems within computer vision became more complex. Independent frame-by-frame analysis is no longer sufficient for analysis of continuous videos.

A variation of LBP that was developed to address the need of a dynamic texture descriptor was volume local binary patterns (VLBP) [32]. VLBP are an extension of LBP into the spatiotemporal domain. VLBP capture dynamic texture by using three parallel frames centered on the current pixel. The need for a dynamic texture descriptor with a lower dimensionality than VLBP inspired the development of local binary patterns in three orthogonal planes (LBP-TOP) [32]. The dimensionality of LBP-TOP is significantly less than VLBP and is computationally less costly than VLBP.

LBP were not always the most popular local appearance feature. Some of the first, most significant works in facial expression analysis by computers used Gabor filters [33]. Gabor filters have historical significance, and they continue to be used in many approaches [34]. Nascent convolutional neural network approaches eventually learn structures similar to a Gabor filter [35]. The Gabor filters are bioinspired and were developed to mimic the V1 cortex of the human visual system. The V1 cortex responds to the gradient images of different orientation and magnitude. It is essentially an appearance-based feature descriptor that

http://dx.doi.org/10.5772/65635

captures all edge information within an image. However, state-of-the-art feature descriptors are known for their compactness and ability to generalize over external and intrinsic factors. The original Gabor filter does not have the ability to generalize in unconstrained settings because it captures all edges within an image, noise included. Furthermore, the Gabor filter is not computationally efficient. The filter produces a response for each filter within its bank. The Gabor filter has been developed into the anisotropic inhibited Gabor filter (AIGF) to model the human visual system's nonclassical receptive field [36]. AIGF generalizes better than the original Gabor filter because of its ability to suppress background noise. A combined Gabor filter with LBP-TOP has been shown to improve accuracy in the classification of facial expressions [37].

A thorough search of literature found no work, which has combined the anisotropic-inhibited Gabor filter and LBP-TOP and this is one of the foci of this chapter. This novel method that compactly encodes the spatiotemporal behavior of a face also removes background texture. It is called *local anisotropic-inhibited binary patterns in three orthogonal planes (LAIBP-TOP).* This feature vector works by first removing all background noise that is captured by the Gabor filter. Only the important edges of the Gabor filter are retained which are then encoded on the *X*, *Y*, and *T* orthogonal planes. The response is succinctly represented as spatiotemporal binary patterns. This feature vector provides a better representation for facial expressions as it is a dynamic texture descriptor and has a smaller feature vector size.

3. Technical approach

Automatic facial emotion recognition by computers has four steps: (1) region-of-interest (ROI) extraction, also known as face detection, (2) registration, colloquially known as alignment, (3) feature extraction, and (4) classification/regression of emotion. This chapter will focus on two important parts of the facial emotion recognition pipeline: face region-of-interest extraction and facial appearance features.

3.1. Reference-based face detection

Reference-based face detection consists of two phases: (1) In the training phase, a reference face is computed with avatar reference image. This face represents a well-extracted face and quantifies the quality of detection results in the next step. (2) In testing, multiple candidate face ROIs are detected, and the candidate ROI that best matches the reference face in the least squared sense is selected for further processing. Three different methodologies for finding the face ROI are combined: a boosted cascade of Haar-like features (Viola and Jones (VJ) [3], a discriminative parameterized appearance model (SIFT landmark points matched with iterative least squares), and a parts-based deformable model. VJ was selected because of its ubiquitous use in the field of face analysis. Discriminative parameterized appearance models were recently deployed in commercial software [38]. Parts-based deformable models showed promise for face ROI extraction in the wild [39]. Despite the success of currently used methods, there is still much room for improvement. In the Motor Trend data, there are segments of video where one extractor will succeed when others fail. Therefore, better performance can be achieved by unifying these three methods to generate multiple candidate face ROIs and quantitatively determine which candidate is the best ROI. Note that Refs. [38, 39] use VJ for an initial bounding box so running more than one face detector is not excessive for state-of-the-art approaches.

3.1.1. *Reference-based face detection in training*

The avatar reference image concept generates a reference image of an expressionless face. It was previously used for registration [40] and learning [41]. A proof of optimality of the avatar image concept is given in the previous work [42]. Let I be an image in the training data D. To estimate the avatar reference image $R_{ARI}(x)$, take the mean across all face images:

$$R_{ARI}(x, y) = \frac{1}{N_D} \sum_{i \in D} I_i(x, y) \quad (1)$$

where N_D is the number of training images; (x, y) is a pixel location; and I_i is the i-th image in the dataset D. The process iterates by rewarping D to R_{ARI} to create a more refined estimate of the reference face. The procedure is described as follows: (1) compute reference using Eq. (1) from all training ROIs D, (2) warp all D to the reference, and (3) recompute Eq. (1) using the warped images from the previous step. Steps (2) and (3) are iterated for three times which was empirically selected in Ref. [40]. Results of the reference face at different iterations are shown in **Figure 1**. SIFT-Flow warps the images in step (2) and the reader is referred to [43] for a full description of SIFT-Flow. In short, a dense, per-pixel SIFT feature warp is computed with loopy belief propagation. After this point, a R_{ARI} represents a well-extracted reference face.

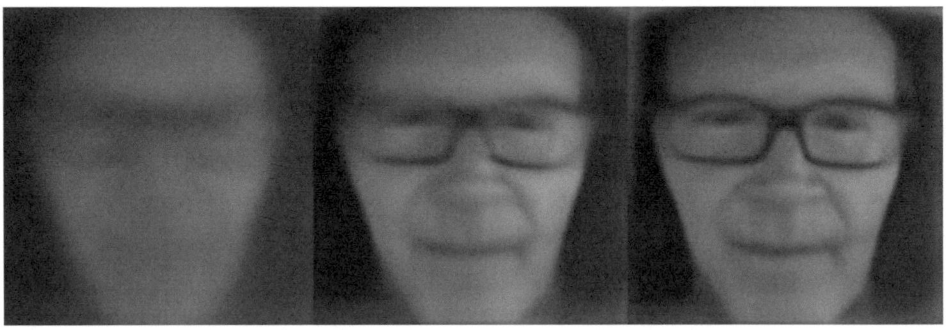

Figure 1. Iterative refinement of the avatar reference face. It represents a well-extracted face.

3.1.2. *Reference-based face detection in testing*

To robustly detect a face, three different pipelines simultaneously extract the ROI. We fuse a discriminative parameterized appearance model, a part-based deformable model, and the

Viola and Jones framework. In Viola and Jones (VJ), detection of the face is carried out with a boosted cascade of Haar-like features. Because of the near-standard use of VJ, we omit an in-depth explanation of the method. The reader is referred to [3] for the details of the algorithm.

3.1.2.1. *Discriminative parameterized appearance model*

Consider a sparse appearance model of the face. The face detection problem can be framed as an optimization problem that fits the landmark points representing the face. A face is successfully detected when the gradient descent in the fitness space of the optimization problem is complete. Traversing the fitness space can be viewed as a supervised learning problem [38], rather than carrying out a gradient descent with Gauss-Newton algorithm [44]. In the training phase the following equation is minimized:

$$\min_{w} \left\| s(p + w(p)) - s(p^{*}) \right\| \tag{2}$$

where s is a function that computes SIFT features; w is a flow vector to be optimized; p^{*} is manually labeled landmark points; and the vector p has horizontal and vertical components $\mathbf{p} = (x, y)$. Computing the Hessian of the model is computationally undesirable, and supervised learning of the descent from p^{*} avoids computing this directly. In testing, face alignment is carried out with linear least squares.

3.1.2.2. *Parts-based deformable models*

Parts-based deformable models represent a face as a collection of landmark points similar to PAMs. The difference is that the most likely locations of the parts are calculated with a probabilistic framework. The landmark points are represented as a mixture of trees of landmark points on the face [39]. Let Φ be the set of landmark points on the face. A facial configuration L is modeled as $L = \{p_i : i \in \Phi\}$. Alignment of the landmark points is achieved by maximizing the posterior likelihood of appearance and shape. The objective function is formulated as follows:

$$\epsilon(I, L, j) = \sum_{i} u_{ij}\, \mathbf{s}(p_i) + \sum_{(i,k)} \left(b_1(i,j,k)\tilde{x}^2 + b_2(i,j,k)\tilde{x} + b_3(i,j,k)\tilde{y}^2 + b_4(i,j,k)\tilde{y} \right) \tag{3}$$

where ϵ is the objective function to be minimized; I is the video frame; j is the mixture index; k is the landmark point indexes; u_{ij} is the template of mixture j at point i; s is an appearance feature; b_1, b_2, b_3, and b_4 are the spring rest and rigidity parameters of the model's shape. $\tilde{x}$ and $\tilde{y}$ are the displacement in horizontal and vertical directions from i and k:

$$\tilde{x} = x_i - x_k \tag{4}$$

$$\tilde{y} = y_i - y_k \tag{5}$$

Inference is carried out by maximizing the following:

$$\max_{j}\left(\max_{L}(\epsilon(I, L, j)) \right) \tag{6}$$

which enumerates over all mixtures and configurations. The maximum likelihood of the model which best fits the parameters is computed with the Chow-Liu algorithm [45].

3.1.2.3. Least square selection

We compare the results of all three pipelines to check if a face has been properly detected. The problem is posed where we must quantify the accuracy of each extraction pipeline. We minimize the candidate face ROI I_k to the reference of a face R_{ARI} in the least squared sense:

$$\min_k \sqrt{\sum p \left(I_k(x, y) - R_{ARI}(x, y)\right)^2} \quad (7)$$

where I_k is a candidate face ROI from one of the face extraction pipelines k. It is possible that Eq. (7) failed to generate a candidate face. There are two causes for this: (A) there are no candidate face ROIs generated, or (B) the selected face is a false alarm, e.g., it is not a face, or the bounding box is poorly centered. To prevent (B), the face selected in Eq. (7) must have a distance to the reference of no greater than parameter T, which is empirically selected in training. If the detector fails because of (A) or the threshold is less than T, the last extracted face should be used for processing further in the recognition pipeline. Note when comparing this proposed method to other detectors in **Table 1** we count (A) and (B) as a failure of the method.

%	Viola and Jones (VJ)	Constrained local models (CLM)	Supervised descent method (SDM)	Proposed face detector
True positive rate	60.27 ± 10.53	68.36 ± 9.80	81.37 ± 17.60	**86.29 ± 8.90**
F1-score	74.52 ± 19.67	80.81 ± 7.17	89.47 ± 11.22	**92.43 ± 5.07**

Viola and Jones is the worst performer with the highest variance. Constrained Local Models and Supervised Descent Method are acceptable but have a high variance. The proposed method is the best performer. Higher is better for both metrics. Bold: Best performer. Underline: Second best performer.

Table 1. Face detection rates for the Motor Trend Magazine's Best Driver Car of the Year.

3.2. Local anisotropic inhibited binary patterns in three orthogonal planes

3.2.1. Gabor filter

A Gabor filter is a bandpass filter that is used for edge detection at a specific orientation and scale. Images are typically filtered by many Gabor filters at different parameters, called a bank. It is modulated by a sine and a cosine. When it is modulated by a sine, the Gabor filter finds symmetric edges. When it is modulated by a cosine, the Gabor filter finds antisymmetric edges. According to Grigorescu et al. [36], a Gabor filter at a specific orientation and magnitude is:

$$g(x, y; \gamma, \theta, \lambda, \sigma, \phi) = \exp\left(\frac{x'^2 + \gamma^2 y'^2}{2\sigma^2}\right)\cos\left(\frac{2\pi x'}{\gamma} + \phi\right) \quad (8)$$

where γ is the spatial aspect ratio that effects the eccentricity of the filter; θ is the angle parameter that tunes the orientation; and λ is the wavelength parameter that tunes the filter to a specific spatial frequency, or magnitude. In pattern recognition this is also referred to a scale. σ is the variance of the distribution. It determines the size of the filter. ϕ is the phase offset that is taken at 0 and π. $x^{'}$ and $y^{'}$ are defined as follows:

$$x^{'} = x\cos\theta + y\sin\theta \tag{9}$$

$$y^{'} = -x\sin\theta + y\cos\theta \tag{10}$$

The Gabor filter can be used as local appearance filter by tuning the filter to a local neighborhood while still varying the orientation: $\sigma/\lambda = 0.56$ and varying θ. For the rest of the chapter, $g(x, y; \theta, \phi)$ represents g with $\gamma = 0.5$, $\lambda = 7.14$, and $\sigma = 3$, and with varying θ and ϕ. Given an image I, the Gabor energy filter is given by:

$$E(x, y; \theta) = \sqrt{\left((I * g)(x, y; \theta, 0)\right)^2 + \left((I * g)(x, y; \theta, \pi)\right)^2} \tag{11}$$

which corresponds to the magnitude of filtering the image at the phase values of 0 and π.

3.2.2. *Anisotropic-inhibited Gabor filter*

The original formulation of the Gabor energy filter does not generalize well. The Gabor energy filter captures all edges and magnitudes within the image, including the edges due to noisy background texture. For example, MPEG block encoding artifacts that present as a grid-like repeating pattern. In the field of facial expression recognition, face morphology causes creases along the face that are not a part of the background texture thus a better contour map can be extracted by removing the background texture of the face. In order to eliminate the background texture detected by the Gabor filter, we build upon the Anisotropic Gabor energy filter. To suppress the background texture, we take a weighted Gabor filter:

$$\tilde{g}(x, y; \theta) = (E * w)(x, y) \tag{12}$$

where the weighted function w is:

$$w(x, y) = \frac{1}{\| DoG(x, y) \|} h(DoG(x, y)) \tag{13}$$

where $h(x) = H(x) * x$, where $H(x)$ is the Heaviside step function; $DoG(.)$ is the difference of Gaussians:

$$DoG(x, y; \theta) = \frac{1}{2\pi K^2 \sigma^2} e^{\frac{x^2+y^2}{2K^2\sigma^2}} - \frac{1}{2\pi\sigma^2} e^{-\frac{x^2+y^2}{2\sigma^2}} \tag{14}$$

w resembles a ring. Eq. (12) retrieves the background texture of (x, y) without the texture of (x, y) itself by weighting E by the ring-like filter w. The resulting anisotropic-inhibited Gabor filter is described as follows:

$$\hat{g}(x, y; \theta) = h(E(x, y; \theta) - \alpha \times \tilde{g}(x, y; \theta)) \tag{15}$$

where α is a parameter that affects how much of the background texture is removed. α ranges from 0 to 1, where 0 indicates no background texture removal and 1 indicates complete background texture removal. The first term of Eq. (15) defines the original Gabor energy filter that captures all edges including background edges. The second term subtracts the weighted

Gabor filter with a specified alpha, depending on how much background suppression is needed. We follow [46] where a value of $\alpha = 1$ was empirically selected.

To obtain an image that contains only the strongest edges and corresponding orientations, we take the edges with the strongest magnitude across N different orientations:

$$AIGF(x, y) = \max_{\theta} \hat{g}(x, y; \theta) \tag{16}$$

The resulting output of Anisotropic Inhibited Gabor Filter is an image that is $M \times N$. Results are given in **Figure 2**.

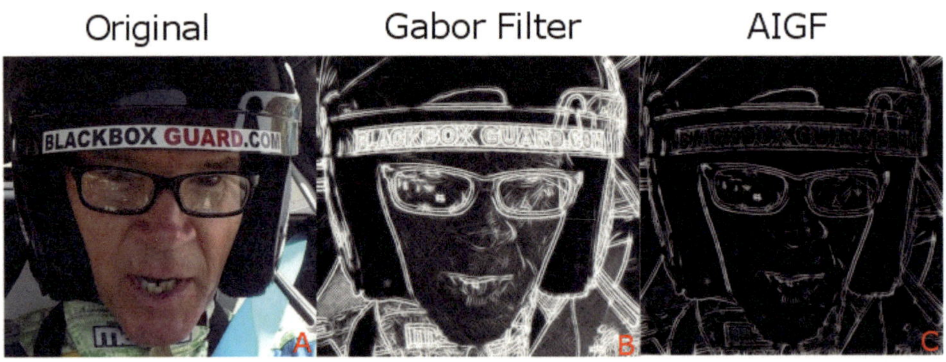

Figure 2. (a) Original frame, (b) result of Gabor energy filter (Eq. (15) with $\alpha = 0$), and (c) result of Anisotropic Gabor Energy Filtering.

We build upon the work in Ref. [46], but the proposed approach is significantly different. The anisotropic Gabor energy filter (AIGF) further computes the orientations corresponding to the maximum edges as follows:

$$\Theta(x, y) = \underset{\theta}{\arg\max}\, \tilde{g}(x, y; \theta) \tag{17}$$

A soft histogram is computed from Θ with votes weighted by the maximal edge response $AIGF$. For the proposed approach, we use $AIGF$ and do not compute a soft histogram.

3.2.3. Local binary patterns

Local binary patterns (LBP) encode local appearance as a microtexture code. The code is a function of comparison to the intensity values of neighboring pixels. Some formulations are invariant to rotation and monotonic grayscale transformations [31]. At present LBP and its many variations are one of the most widely used feature descriptors for facial expression recognition. LBP result in a texture descriptor with dimensionality of 2^n where n is a parameter that controls the number of pixel neighbours. The LBP code of a pixel at (x, y) is given as follows:

$$LBP(x, y) = \sum_{\{u,v\} \in N_{x,y}^{LBP}} \mathrm{sign}(I(u, v) - I(x, y)) \times 2^q \tag{18}$$

where (u, v) iterates over points in the neighborhood of $N_{x,y}^{LBP}$; $\mathrm{sign}(.)$ is the sign of the expression; q is a counter starting from 0 that increments on each iteration; and $N_{x,y}^{LBP}$ is the neighborhood of points about (x, y) (see **Figure 3A**). 2^q encodes the result of the intensity difference in a specific bit. A histogram is taken for further compactness and tolerance of registration errors. Each pixel in I is encoded with an LBP code from Eq. (18) then an n-level histogram is extracted from LBP. Typically, the image is segmented into nonoverlapping regions and a histogram is extracted from each region [47]. While powerful and effective for static images, LBP lacks the ability to capture temporal changes in continuous video data.

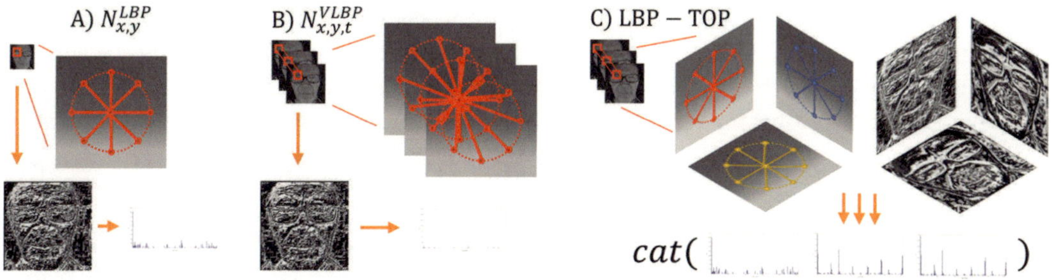

Figure 3. (A) In LBP, microtexture is encoded in the XY-plane. (B) In VLBP, this is extended to the spatiotemporal domain by including neighbors in the three planes parallel to the current frame. (C) In LBP-TOP, local binary patterns are separately extracted in three orthogonal planes and the resultant histograms are concatenated. This greatly reduces feature vector size over treating the volume as a 3D microtexture.

3.2.4. *Volumetric local binary patterns*

Volume local binary patterns (VLBP) and local binary patterns in three orthogonal planes (LBP-TOP) are variations of LBP that were developed to capture dynamic textures for video data. In VLBP, the circle of neighboring points in LBP is scaled up to a cylinder. VLBP computes code values as a function of three parallel planes centered at $\{x, y, t\}$. That is, the middle plane contains the center pixel. VLBP coding is obtained by the following equation:

$$VLBP(x, y, t) = \sum_{k \in \{-L,0,L\}} \sum_{\{u,v\} \in N_{x,y,t}^{VLBP}} \text{sign}(I(u, v, k) - I(x, y, t)) \times 2^q \quad (19)$$

where k iterates over three time points: t, $t-L$, and $t+L$. $N_{x,y,t}^{VLBP}$ is the set of spatiotemporal neighbours of $\{x, y, t\}$ (see **Figure 3B**). A large set of $N_{x,y,t}^{VLBP}$ results in a large feature vector while a small $N_{x,y,t}^{VLBP}$ results in a small feature vector. As with LBP, a histogram is taken for further compactness. The maximum grey-level from Eq. (19) is $2^{(3n+2)}$, thus VLBP are more computationally expensive to calculate and require larger feature vector.

3.2.5. *Local binary patterns in three orthogonal planes*

LBP-TOP was developed as an alternative to VLBP. VLBP and LBP-TOP differ in two ways. First, LBP-TOP uses three orthogonal planes that intersect at the center pixel. Second, VLBP considers the cooccurrences of all neighboring points from three parallel frames, which make for a larger feature vector. LBP-TOP only considers features from each separate plane and then concatenates them together, making the feature vector much shorter when compared to VLBP for large values of n. LBP-TOP performs LBP on the three orthogonal planes corresponding to the XY, XT, and YT axes (see **Figure 3C**). The XY plane contributes the spatial information and the *XT* and *YT* frames contribute the temporal information. These planes intersect at the center pixel. Whereas in Eq. (19), VLBP captures a truly three- dimensional microtexture, LBP-TOP computes LBP codes separately on each plane. The resulting feature vector dimensionality of LBP-TOP is 3×2^n.

3.2.6. Local anisotropic inhibited Gabor patterns in three orthogonal planes

In the proposed method, the computational efficiency of LBP-TOP is applied to images filtered with the anisotropic-inhibited Gabor filter. The suppression of background texture provides an image that only contains the edges separate from the background texture. These edges are the significant boundaries of facial features that are useful when determining expression and emotion. Local anisotropic binary patterns' (LAIBP) code values are computed as follows:

$$LAIBP(x, y) = \sum_{\{u,v\} \in N_{x,y}^{LBP}} \text{sign}\big(AIGF(u, v) - AIGF(x, y)\big) \times 2^q \tag{20}$$

where $g(u, v)$ is the maximal edge magnitude from Eq. (16). LAIBP-TOP features are extracted in a similar fashion to LBP-TOP: Compute *LAIBP* codes from Eq. (20) in *XY*, *XT*, and *YT* planes and concatenate the resultant histograms. A comparison of AIGF, LBP, and the proposed method, LAIBP, are given in **Figure 4**. The proposed method (LAIBP-TOP) is significantly different from LBP-TOP because we introduce background texture removal from Eq. (16).

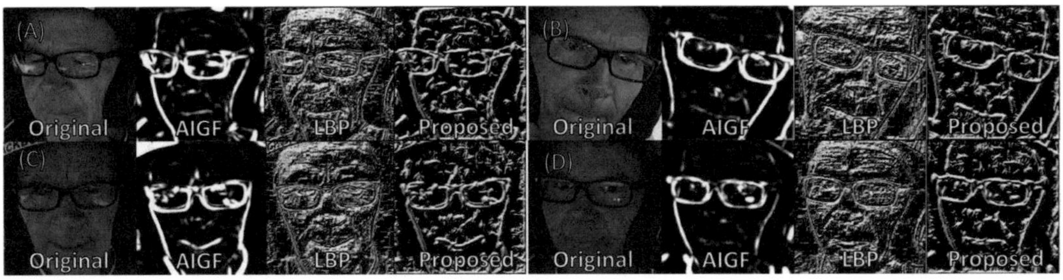

Figure 4. From left to right: The original frame, anisotropic inhibited Gabor filter (AIGF), local binary patterns (LBP), and the proposed method local anisotropic inhibited binary patterns (LAIBP). Note that the proposed method has more continuous lines compared to AIGF. LBP is susceptible to JPEG compression artifacts.

4. Experimental results

4.1. Datasets

Data in this work have been provided by Motor Trend Magazine from their Best Driver Car of the Year 2014 and 2015. They consist of frontal face video of a test driver as he drives one of 10 automobiles around a racetrack. Parts of the video will be released publicly on YouTube at a later date. The videos are 1080p HD quality captured with a Go Pro Hero 4 and range from 231 to 720 seconds in length. The camera is mounted on the windshield of the car facing the driver's face. The dataset was labeled with the Fontaine emotional model [2] rather than facial action units or emotional categories to quantize emotion. Emotions such as happiness, sadness, etc. occupy a space in a two-dimensional Euclidean space defined by valence and arousal. The objective of the dataset is to detect the valence and arousal of an individual on a per-frame basis. Valence, also known as evaluation-pleasantness, describes positivity or negativity of the person's feelings or feelings of situation, e.g., happiness versus sadness. Arousal, also known as activation-arousal, describes a person's interest in the situation, e.g., eagerness versus anxiety.

4.2. Metrics

For face detection results, we use true positive rate and F_1 score. F_1 score is given by:

$$2 \times \frac{(\text{Precision})(\text{Recall})}{(\text{Precision}) + (\text{Recall})} \tag{21}$$

For both metrics, higher is better. For full recognition results, we use root mean squared (RMS) error and correlation. The correlation coefficient is given by:

$$\frac{E\left[\left(y_d - \mu_{y_d}\right)\left(y - \mu_y\right)\right]}{\sigma_{y_d}\sigma_y} \tag{22}$$

where $E[.]$ is the expected operation; y_d is the vector of ground-truth labels for a video; y is the vector of predicted labels for a video; μ_{y_d} and μ_y are the mean of ground-truth and prediction, respectively; and σ_{y_d} and σ_y are the standard deviation of ground-truth and prediction, respectively.

4.3. Results comparing different face detectors

Face detection results are given in **Table 1**. In general, VJ is the worst performer with the highest variance. Though CLM and SDM have acceptable detection rates, they too have a high variance and some videos are a total failure with no face extraction. The proposed algorithm improves detection rates on both datasets and reduces variance.

4.4. Results comparing different facial appearance features

For the full recognition pipeline: The landmarks for the inner corner of the eyes and the tip of the nose are used as control points for a course registration. These points are the least effected by face morphology. An ϵ-SVR is used for prediction of valence and arousal values [48].

Full regression results and a comparison to other state-of-the-art facial appearance features are given in **Table 2**. Experiments employed a 9-fold, leave-one-video-out cross-validation. For correlation, higher is better; for RMS lower is better. In **Table 2**, the correlation and RMS values for valence and arousal labels by the proposed method performed the best for valence and second best for arousal. Removal of background noise and then implementing LBP-TOP provided better results. RMS values for the proposed method are also the best for arousal and second best for valence. The proposed method has the best average correlation and the lowest average RMS value. Graphs comparing the ground-truth and predicted labels are given in **Figure 5**. It was found that frames with extreme head rotation tended to have lower correlation and higher error due to the difficulty of registering the dataset.

Features	Valence		Arousal		Average	
	Correlation	RMS	Correlation	RMS	Correlation	RMS
LBP	0.0066	0.5025	0.1032	0.2526	0.0549	0.3776
VLBP	0.3060	**0.1292**	**0.3810**	0.2428	0.3435	0.1860
LBP-TOP	0.3705	0.2134	0.0819	0.1624	0.2262	0.1879
Gaborenergy filter	0.1296	0.3937	0.0569	0.1935	0.0933	0.2936
LGBP-TOP	0.2805	1.1207	0.0787	1.2559	0.1796	1.1883
Proposed	**0.4446**	0.2054	0.2801	**0.1547**	**0.3624**	**0.1801**

Note: The proposed method has better average correlation for valence and arousal. Bold indicates best performing feature.

Table 2. Correlation and RMS for prediction of valence and arousal emotion categories on the Motor Trend Magazine Best Driver's Car of the Year.

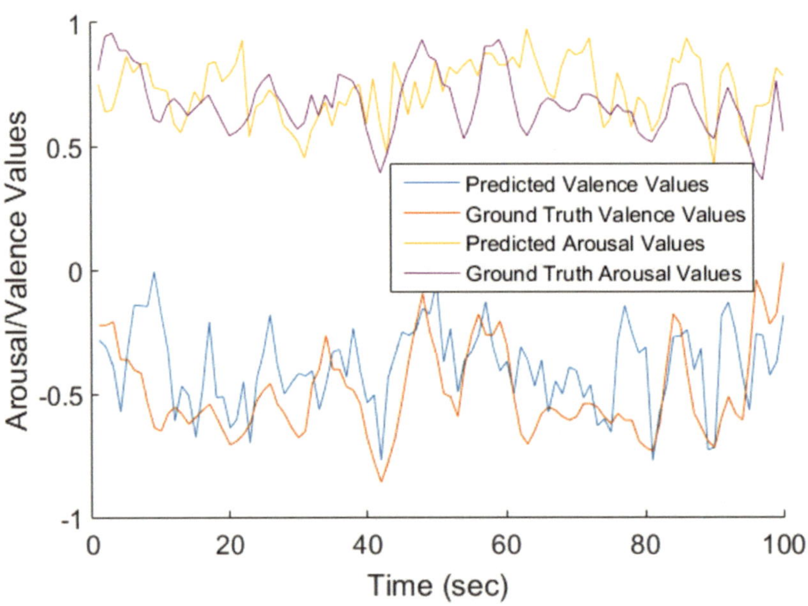

Figure 5. The predicted values are graphed with the values for valence and arousal.

5. Conclusions

In this chapter, we proposed a system to perform facial expression recognition on a brand new dataset. This dataset is unconstrained and unique. We proposed a new feature vector that is robust to background noise and capable of capturing dynamic textures. We also proposed a novel method for fusing the output of many face detectors. Both approaches provided better results than other state-of-the-art methods. In the future work, the face detection scheme will be scaled up to a 3D model to better detect the extreme out of plane head rotations.

Author details

Albert C. Cruz[1]*, Bir Bhanu[2] and Belinda T. Le[2]

*Address all correspondence to: acruz37@csub.edu

1 COMputer Perception LAB (COMPLAB), California State University, Bakersfield, CA, USA

2 Center for Research in Intelligent Systems (CRIS), University of California, Riverside, CA, USA

References

[1] K. Reynolds, "At 2015 Best Driver's Car, What is the Driver Experiencing?," *Motor Trend Magazine*, 2015. [Online]. Available: http://www.motortrend.com/news/the-future-of-testing-measuring-the-driver-as-well-as-the-car/. [Accessed: 26-Apr-2016].

[2] J. R. J. Fontaine, K. R. Scherer, E. B. Roesch, and P. C. Ellsworth, "The world of emotions is not two-dimensional," *Psychol. Sci.*, vol. 18, no. 12, pp. 1050–1057, 2007.

[3] P. Viola and M. Jones, "Rapid object detection using a boosted cascade of simple features," *Proc. 2001 IEEE Comput. Soc. Conf. Comput. Vis. Pattern Recognition. CVPR 2001*, vol. 1, 2001.

[4] J. White, C. Thompson, H. Turner, B. Dougherty, and D. C. Schmidt, "WreckWatch: Automatic traffic accident detection and notification with smartphones," *Mob. Networks Appl.*, vol. 16, no. 3, pp. 285–303, 2011.

[5] S. Echegaray, "The modular design and implementation of an intelligent cruise control system," in *2008 IEEE International Conference on System of Systems Engineering*, 2008, pp. 1–6.

[6] R. C. Coetzer and G. P. Hancke, "Eye detection for a real-time vehicle driver fatigue monitoring system," in *IEEE Intelligent Vehicles Symposium, Proceedings*, 2011, pp. 66–71.

[7] J. L. Gabbard, G. M. Fitch, and H. Kim, "Behind the glass: Driver challenges and opportunities for AR automotive applications," *Proc. IEEE*, vol. 102, no. 2, pp. 124–136, 2014.

[8] C. Darwin, "The expression of the emotions in man and animals," *Am. J. Med. Sci.*, vol. 232, no. 4, p. 477, 1872.

[9] F. I. Parke, "A model for human faces that allows speech synchronized animation," *Comput. Graph.*, vol. 1, no. 1, pp. 3–4, 1975.

[10] H. Meng, D. Huang, H. Wang, H. Yang, M. AI-Shuraifi, and Y. Wang, "Depression recognition based on dynamic facial and vocal expression features using partial least square regression," in *Avec '13*, 2013, pp. 21–30.

[11] M. Kächele and M. Schels, "Inferring depression and affect from application dependent meta knowledge," in *ACM Multimedia Workshops*, 2014, pp. 41–48.

[12] J. F. Cohn, T. S. Kruez, I. Matthews, Y. Yang, M. H. Nguyen, M. T. Padilla, F. Zhou, and F. De La Torre, "Detecting depression from facial actions and vocal prosody," in *Proceedings—2009 3rd International Conference on Affective Computing and Intelligent Interaction and Workshops, ACII 2009*, 2009.

[13] S. Yang and M. Kafai, "Zapping Index: using smile to measure advertisement zapping likelihood," *IEEE Trans. Affect. Comput.*, vol. 5, no. 4, pp. 432–444, 2014.

[14] S. Demyanov, C. Leckie, and J. Bailey, "Detection of deception in the mafia party game," in *ACM International Conf. Multimedia*, 2015, pp. 335–342.

[15] R. Mihalcea and M. Burzo, "Towards multimodal deception detection – step 1: building a collection of deceptive videos," *ACM Int. Conf. Multimodal Interact.*, pp. 189–192, 2012.

[16] T. O. Meservy, M. L. Jensen, J. Kruse, J. K. Burgoon, J. F. Nunamaker, D. P. Twitchell, G. Tsechpenakis, and D. N. Metaxas, "Deception detection through automatic, unobtrusive analysis of nonverbal behavior," *IEEE Intell. Syst.*, vol. 20, no. 5, pp. 36–43, 2005.

[17] P. Fletcher, "Automobile driver attention indicator," US 3227998 A, 1966.

[18] Y. Wang, B. Reimer, J. Dobres, and B. Mehler, "The sensitivity of different methodologies for characterizing drivers' gaze concentration under increased cognitive demand," *Transp. Res. Part F Traffic Psychol. Behav.*, vol. 26, no. PA, pp. 227–237, 2014.

[19] N. Merat, A. H. Jamson, F. C. H. Lai, M. Daly, and O. M. J. Carsten, "Transition to manual: Driver behaviour when resuming control from a highly automated vehicle," *Transp. Res. Part F Traffic Psychol. Behav.*, vol. 27, no. PB, pp. 274–282, 2014.

[20] A. Tawari, S. Sivaraman, M. M. Trivedi, T. Shannon, and M. Tippelhofer, "Looking-in and looking-out vision for Urban Intelligent Assistance: Estimation of driver attentive state and dynamic surround for safe merging and braking," *IEEE Intell. Veh. Symp. Proc.*, no. Iv, pp. 115–120, 2014.

[21] A. Tawari, S. Martin, and M. M. Trivedi, "Continuous head movement estimator for driver assistance: Issues, algorithms, and on-road evaluations," *IEEE Trans. Intell. Transp. Syst.*, vol. 15, no. 2, pp. 818–830, 2014.

[22] K. Reynolds, "2014 motor trend's best driver's car: How we test," *Motor Trend Magazine*, 2014.

[23] F. De Torre and M. H. Nguyen, "Parameterized kernel principal component analysis: Theory and applications to supervised and unsupervised image alignment," in *IEEE Conf. Computer Vision and Pattern Recognition*, 2008.

[24] A. Savran, H. Cao, M. Shah, A. Nenkova, and R. Verma, "Combining video, audio and lexical indicators of affect in spontaneous conversation via particle filtering," *ICMI'12—Proc. ACM Int. Conf. Multimodal Interact.*, no. Section 4, pp. 485–492, 2012.

[25] A. Cruz, B. Bhanu, and N. Thakoor, "Facial emotion recognition in continuous video," *Int. Conf. Pattern Recognit.*, pp. 1880–1883, 2012.

[26] J. R. Williamson, W. Street, T. F. Quatieri, B. S. Helfer, R. Horwitz, and B. Yu, "Vocal biomarkers of depression based on motor incoordination and timing," in *ACM International Workshop on Audio/Visual Emotion Challenge*, 2014, pp. 41–47.

[27] G. A. Ramirez, T. Baltrušaitis, and L. P. Morency, "Modeling latent discriminative dynamic of multi-dimensional affective signals," in *Affective Computing and Intelligent Interaction Workshops*, 2011, vol. 6975, pp. 396–406.

[28] P. Dollár, P. Welinder, and P. Perona, "Cascaded pose regression," in *IEEE Conf. Computer Vision and Pattern Recognition*, 2010, pp. 1078–1085.

[29] E. Sanchez-Lozano, F. De la Torre, and D. Gonzalez-Jimenez, "Continuous regression for non-rigid image alignment," in *European Conf. Computer Vision*, 2012, pp. 250–263.

[30] T. F. Cootes, M. C. Ionita, C. Lindner, and P. Sauer, "Robust and accurate shape model fitting using random forest regression voting," in *European Conf. Computer Vision*, 2012, pp. 278–291.

[31] T. Ojala, M. Pietikäinen, and D. Harwood, "A comparative study of texture measures with classification based on featured distributions," *Pattern Recognit.*, vol. 29, no. 1, pp. 51–59, 1996.

[32] G. Zhao and M. Pietikäinen, "Dynamic texture recognition using volume local binary patterns," *Proc. ECCV 2006 Work. Dyn. Vis.*, vol. 4358, pp. 165–177, 2006.

[33] M. Lyons, S. Akamatsu, M. Kamachi, and J. Gyoba, "Coding facial expressions with Gabor wavelets," in *Proceedings—3rd IEEE International Conference on Automatic Face and Gesture Recognition, FG 1998*, 1998, pp. 200–205.

[34] F. Ringeval, M. Valstar, E. Marchi, D. Lalanne, and R. Cowie, "The AV + EC 2015 multimodal affect recognition challenge: Bridging across audio, video, and physiological data categories and subject descriptors," in *Proc. ACM Multimedia Workshops*, 2015.

[35] J. Yosinski, J. Clune, Y. Bengio, and H. Lipson, "How transferable are features in deep neural networks?," *Adv. Neural Inf. Process. Syst. 27 (Proceedings NIPS)*, vol. 27, pp. 1–9, 2014.

[36] C. Grigorescu, N. Petkov, and M. A. Westenberg, "Contour detection based on nonclassical receptive field inhibition," *IEEE Trans. Image Process.*, vol. 12, no. 7, pp. 729–739, 2003.

[37] T. R. Almaev and M. F. Valstar, "Local gabor binary patterns from three orthogonal planes for automatic facial expression recognition," *Proc.—2013 Hum. Assoc. Conf. Affect. Comput. Intell. Interact. ACII 2013*, pp. 356–361, 2013.

[38] X. Xiong and F. De La Torre, "Supervised descent method and its applications to face alignment," in *Proc. Conf. on Computer Vision and Pattern Recognition*, 2013, pp. 532–539.

[39] S. Cheng, A. Asthana, S. Zafeiriou, J. Shen, and M. Pantic, "Real-time generic face tracking in the wild with CUDA," *Proc. 5th ACM Multimed. Syst. Conf. - MMSys '14*, no. 1, pp. 148–151, 2014.

[40] S. Yang and B. Bhanu, "Understanding discrete facial expressions in video using an emotion avatar image," *IEEE Trans. Syst. Man, Cybern. Part B Cybern.*, vol. 42, no. 4, pp. 980–992, 2012.

[41] A. C. Cruz, B. Bhanu, and N. Thakoor, "Facial emotion recognition with expression energy," *ACM Int'l. Conf. Multimodal Interact. Work.*, pp. 457–464, 2012.

[42] E. Cambria, G.-B. Huang, L. L. C. Kasun, H. Zhou, C. M. Vong, J. Lin, J. Yin, Z. Cai, Q. Liu, K. Li, V. C. M. Leung, L. Feng, Y.-S. Ong, M.-H. Lim, A. Akusok, A. Lendasse, F. Corona, R. Nian, Y. Miche, P. Gastaldo, R. Zunino, S. Decherchi, X. Yang, K. Mao, B.-S. Oh, J. Jeon, K.-A. Toh, A. B. J. Teoh, J. Kim, H. Yu, Y. Chen, and J. Liu, "Extreme learning machines [trends & controversies]," *IEEE Intell. Syst.*, vol. 28, no. 6, pp. 30–59, 2013.

[43] C. Liu, J. Yuen, and A. Torralba, "Sift flow: Dense correspondence across scenes and its applications," *IEEE Trans. Pattern Anal. Mach. Intell.*, vol. 33, no. 5, pp. 15–49, 2015.

[44] S. Baker and I. Matthews, "Lucas-Kanade 20 years on: A unifying framework," *Int. J. Comput. Vis.*, vol. 56, no. 3, pp. 221–255, 2004.

[45] C. Chow and C. Liu, "Discrete probability distributions with dependence trees," *IEEE Trans. Inf. Theory*, vol. 14, no. 3, pp. 462–467, 1968.

[46] A. C. Cruz, B. Bhanu, and N. S. Thakoor, "Background suppressing Gabor energy filtering," *Pattern Recognit. Lett.*, vol. 52, pp. 40–47, 2015.

[47] A. Cruz, B. Bhanu, and N. Thakoor, "Vision and attention theory based sampling for continuous facial emotion recognition," *IEEE Trans. Affect. Comput.*, vol. PP, no. 99, pp. 1–1, 2014.

[48] C.-C. Chang and C.-J. Lin, "LIBSVM," *ACM Trans. Intell. Syst. Technol.*, vol. 2, no. 3, pp. 1–27, 2011.

Chapter 3

Affective Valence Detection from EEG Signals Using Wrapper Methods

Antonio R. Hidalgo-Muñoz, Míriam M. López,
Isabel M. Santos, Manuel Vázquez-Marrufo,
Elmar W. Lang and Ana M. Tomé

Additional information is available at the end of the chapter

http://dx.doi.org/10.5772/66667

Abstract

In this work, a novel valence recognition system applied to EEG signals is presented. It consists of a feature extraction block followed by a wrapper classification algorithm. The proposed feature extraction method is based on measures of relative energies computed in short-time intervals and certain frequency bands of EEG signal segments time-locked to the stimuli presentation. These measures represent event-related desynchronization/synchronization of underlying brain neural networks. The subsequent feature selection and classification steps comprise a wrapper technique based on two different classification approaches: an ensemble classifier, i.e., a random forest of classification trees and a support vector machine algorithm. Applying a proper importance measure from the classifiers, the feature elimination has been used to identify the most relevant features of the decision making both for intrasubject and intersubject settings, using single trial signals and ensemble averaged signals, respectively. The proposed methodologies allowed us to identify a frontal region and a beta band as the most relevant characteristics, extracted from the electrical brain activity, in order to determine the affective valence elicited by visual stimuli.

Keywords: EEG, random forest, SVM, wrapper method

1. Introduction

During the last decade, information about the emotional state of users has become more and more important in computer-based technologies. Several emotion recognition methods and their applications have been addressed, including facial expression and microexpression recognition, vocal feature recognition and electrophysiology-based systems [1]. More recently, the integration of emotion forecasting systems in ambient-assistant living paradigms has been considered [2]. Concerning the origin of the signal sources, the used signals can be divided into two categories: those originating from the peripheral nervous system (e.g., heart rate, electromyogram, galvanic skin resistance, etc.) and those originating from the central nervous system (e.g., electroencephalogram (EEG)). Traditionally, EEG-based technology has been used in medical applications but nowadays it is spreading to other areas such as entertainment [3] and brain-computer interfaces (BCI) [4]. With the emergence of wearable and portable devices, a vast amount of digital data are produced and there is an increasing interest in the development of machine-learning software applications using EEG signals. For the efficient manipulation of this high-dimensional data, various soft computing paradigms have been introduced either for feature extraction or pattern recognition tasks. Nevertheless, up to now, as far as authors are aware, few research works have focused on the criteria to select the most relevant features linked to emotions, relying most of the studies on basic statistics.

It is not easy to compare different emotion recognition systems, since they differ in the way emotions are elicited and in the underlying model of emotions (e.g., discrete or dimensional model of emotions) [5]. According to the dimensional model of emotions, psychologists represent emotions in a 2D valence/arousal space [6]. While valence refers to the pleasure or displeasure that a stimulus causes, arousal refers to the alertness level which is elicited by the stimulus (see **Figure 1**). Sometimes an additional category assigned as *neutral* is included, which is represented in the region close to the origin of the 2D valence/arousal space. Some studies concentrate on one of the dimensions of the space such as identifying the arousal intensity or the valence (low/negative versus high/positive) and eventually a third class neutral state. Recently, it was pointed out that data analysis competitions, similar to the brain-computer interfaces community, could encourage the researchers to disseminate and compare their methodologies [7].

Normally, emotions can be elicited by different procedures, for instance by presenting an external stimulus (picture, sound, word, or video), by facing a concrete interaction or situation [8] or by simply asking subjects to imagine different kinds of emotions. Concerning external visual stimuli, one may resort to standard databases such as the international affective picture system (IAPS) collection which is widely used [7, 9] or the DEAP database [10] that also includes some physiological signals recorded during multimedia stimuli presentation. Similar to any other classification system, in physiology-based recognition systems, it is needed to establish which signals will be used to extract relevant features from these input signals and finally to use them for training a classifier. However, as often it occurs in many biomedical data applications, the initial feature vector dimension can be very large in comparison to the number of examples to train (and evaluate) the classifier.

In this work, we prove the suitability of incorporating a wrapper strategy for feature elimination to improve the classification accuracy and to identify the most relevant EEG features (according to the standard 10/20 system). We propose it by using the spectral features related to EEG synchronization, which has never been applied before for similar purposes. Two learning algorithms integrating the classification block are compared: random forest and support vector machine (SVM). In addition, our automatic valence recognition system has been tested both in intra and intersubject modalities, whose input signals are single trials (segments of signal after the stimulus presentation) of only one participant and ensemble averaged signals computed for each stimulus category and every participant, respectively.

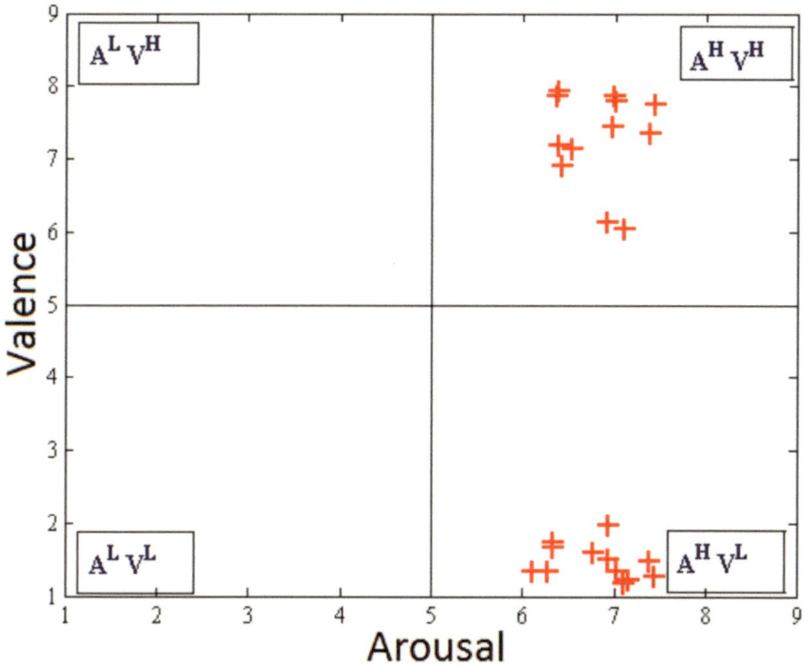

Figure 1. Ratings of the pictures selected from international affective picture system for carrying out the experiment. L: low rating; H: high rating.

2. Related work

The following subsections review some examples of machine learning approaches to affective computing and brain cognitive works where time-domain and frequency-domain signal features are related to the processing of emotions.

2.1. Classification systems and emotion

The pioneering work of Picard [11] on affective computing reports a recognition rate of 81%, achieved by collecting blood pressure, skin conductance and respiration information from one person during several weeks. The subject, an experienced actor, tried to express eight affective states with the aid of a computer-controlled prompting system. In Ref. [12], using the IAPS data set as stimulus repertoire, peripheral biological signals were collected from a single person during several days and at different times of the day. By using a neural network classifier, they considered that the estimation of the valence value (63.8%) is a much harder task than the estimation of arousal (89.3%). In Ref. [13], a study with 50 participants, aged from 7 to

8 years old, is presented. The visual stimulation with the IAPS data set was considered insufficient, hence they proposed a sophisticated scenario to elicit emotions and only peripheral biological signals were recorded and the measured features were the input of a classification scheme based on an SVM. The results showed accuracies of 78.4% and 61% for three and four different categories of emotions, respectively.

In Ref. [14], also by means of the IAPS repository, three emotional states were induced in five male participants: *pleasant*, *neutral* and *unpleasant*. They obtained, using SVMs, an accuracy of 66.7% for these three classes of emotion, solely based on features extracted from EEG signals. A similar strategy was followed by Macas [15], where the EEG data were collected from 23 subjects during an affective picture stimulus presentation to induce four emotional states in arousal/valence space. The automatic recognition of the individual emotional states was performed with a Bayes classifier. The mean accuracy of the individual classification was about 75%.

In Ref. [16], four emotional categories of the arousal/valence space were considered and the EEG was recorded from 28 participants. The ensemble average signals were computed for each stimulus category and person. Several characteristics (peaks and latencies) as well as frequency-related features (event-related synchronization) were measured on a signal ensemble encompassing three channels located along the anterior-posterior line. Then, a classifier (a decision tree, C4.5 algorithm) was applied to the set of features to identify the affective state. An average accuracy of 77.7% was reported.

In Ref. [17], through a series of projections of facial expression images, emotions were elicited. EEG signals were collected from 16 healthy subjects using only three frontal EEG channels. In Ref. [18], four different classifiers (quadratic discriminant analysis (QDA), k-nearest neighbor (KNN), Mahalanobis distance and SVMs) were implemented in order to accomplish the emotion recognition. For the single channel case, the best results were obtained by the QDA (62.3% mean classification rate), whereas for the combined channel case, the best results were obtained using SVM (83.33% mean classification rate), for the hardest case of differentiating six basic discrete emotions.

In Ref. [19], *IF-THEN* rules of a neurofuzzy system detecting positive and negative emotions are discussed. The study presents the individual performance (ranging from 60 to 82%) of the system for the recognition of emotions (two or four categories) of 11 participants. The decision process is organized into levels where fuzzy membership functions are calculated and combined to achieve decisions about emotional states. The inputs of the system are not only EEG-based features, but also visual features computed on the presented stimulus image.

2.2. Event-related potentials and emotion

Studies of event-related potentials (ERPs) deal with signals that can be tackled at different levels of analysis: signals from single-trials, ensemble averaged signals where the ensemble encompasses several single-trials and signals resulting from a grand-average over different trials as well as subjects. The segments of the time series containing the single-trial response signals are time-locked with the stimulus: t_i (negative value) before and t_f (positive value) after stimulus onset. The ensemble average, over trials of one subject, eliminates the spontaneous activity of brain and the spurious noisy contributions, maintaining only the activity that is phase-locked with the stimulus onset. The grand-average is the average, over participants, of ensemble averages and it is used mostly for visualization purposes to illustrate the outcomes of the study. Usually, a large number of epochs linked to the same stimulus type need to be averaged in order to enhance the signal-to-noise ratio (SNR) and to keep the mentioned phase-locked contribution of the ERP. Experimental psychology studies on emotions show that the ERPs have characteristics (amplitude and latency) of the early waves which change according to the nature of the stimuli [20, 21]. In Ref. [16], the characteristics of ensemble-average are the features of the classifier. However, this model can only roughly approximate reality, since it cannot deal with robust dynamical changes that occur in the human brain [22].

Due to the mentioned limitation, frequency analysis is more appropriate, as long as it is assumed that certain events affect specific bands of the ongoing EEG activity. Therefore, several investigations have studied the effect of stimuli on characteristic frequency bands. Hence, these measures reflect changes in gamma (γ), beta (β), alpha (α), theta (θ) or delta (δ) bands and can be used as input to a classification system. It is known that beta waves are connected to an alert state of mind, whereas alpha waves are more dominant in a relaxing context [23]. Alpha waves are also typically linked to expectancy phenomena and it has been suggested that the main sources of them are located in parietal areas, while beta activity is most prominent in the frontal cortex over other areas during intense-focused mental activity [22]. Furthermore, regarding the emotional valence processing, psychophysiological research works have shown different patterns in the electrical activity recorded from the two hemispheres [24]. By comparing the power of spectral bands between the left and the right hemisphere of the brain of one participant, they reveal that the left frontal area is related to positive valence, whereas the right one is more related to negative valence [25].

In brain-related studies, one of the most popular, a simple and reliable measure from the spectral domain is the event-related desychronization/synchronization (ERD/ERS). It represents a relative decrease (ERD) or increase (ERS) in the power content in time intervals after the stimulus onset when compared to a reference interval defined before the stimulus onset [26]. ERD/ERS estimated for the relevant frequency bands during the perception of emotional stimulus have been analyzed [27, 28]. It is suggested that ERS in the theta band is related to emotional processes, together with an interaction between valence and hemisphere for the anterior-temporal regions [27]. Later on, experiments showed that the degree of emotional impact of the stimulus is significantly associated with increase in evoked synchronization in the δ-, α-, β-, γ- bands [28]. In the same study, it was also suggested that the anterior areas of the cortex of both hemispheres are associated predominantly with the valence dimension of emotion. Moreover, in Ref. [29], it has been suggested that delta and theta bands are involved in distinguishing between emotional and neutral states, either with explicit or implicit emotions. Furthermore, in Ref. [30], the results showed that centrofrontal areas showed significant differences of ERD-delta associated with the valence dimension. They also reported that desynchronization of the medium alpha range is associated with attentional resources. More recently, in Ref. [31], the relationships of the late positive potential (LPP) and alpha-ERD during the viewing of emotional pictures have been investigated. The statistical results obtained by these studies show that it is worth considering ERD/ERS measures as inputs to classifiers meant to automatically recognize emotions. Interestingly, a recent review about affective computing systems [7] emphasizes the advantages of using frequency-based features instead of the ERP components.

3. Materials and methods

In our valence detection system, we have addressed the problem of selecting the most relevant features to define the scalp region of interest by including a wrapper-based classification block. Feature extraction is based on ERD/ERS measures computed in short intervals and is performed either on signals averaged over an ensemble of trials or on single-trial response signals, in order to carry out inter and intrasubject analysis, respectively. The subsequent wrapper classification stage is implemented using two different classifiers: an ensemble classifier, i.e., a random forest and an SVM. The feature selection of algorithm is wrapped around the classification of algorithm recursively identifying the features which do not contribute to the decision. These features are eliminated from the feature vector. This goal is achieved by applying an importance measure, which depends on the parameters of the classifier. The two variants of the system were implemented in MATLAB also using some facilities of open source software tools like EEGLAB [32], as well as random forest and SVM packages [33].

3.1. Data set

A total of 26 female volunteers participated in the study (age 18-62 years; mean = 24.19; SD = 10.46). Only adult women were chosen in this experiment to avoid gender differences [21, 34, 35]. All participants had normal or corrected to normal vision and none of them had a history of severe medical treatment, neither psychological nor neurological disorders. This study was carried out in compliance with the Helsinki Declaration and its protocol was approved by the Department of Education from the University of Aveiro. All participants signed informed consents before their inclusion.

Each one of the selected participants was comfortably seated at 70 cm from a computer screen (43.2 cm), alone in an enclosed room. The volunteer was instructed verbally to watch some pictures, which appeared on the center of the screen and to stay quiet. No responses were required. The pictures were chosen from the IAPS repository. A total of 24 images with high arousal ratings (>6) were selected, 12 of them with positive affective valence (7.29 ± 0.65) and the other 12 with negative affective valence (1.47 ± 0.24). In order to match as closely as possible the levels of arousal between positive and negative valence stimuli, only high arousal pictures were shown, avoiding neutral pictures. **Figure 1** shows the representation of the stimuli in arousal/valence space.

Three blocks with the same 24 images were presented consecutively and pictures belonging to each block were presented in a pseudorandom order. In each trial, a fixation single cross was presented on the center of the screen during 750 ms, after which an image was presented during 500 ms and finally, a black screen during 2250 ms (total duration = 3500 ms). **Figure 2** shows a scheme of the experimental protocol.

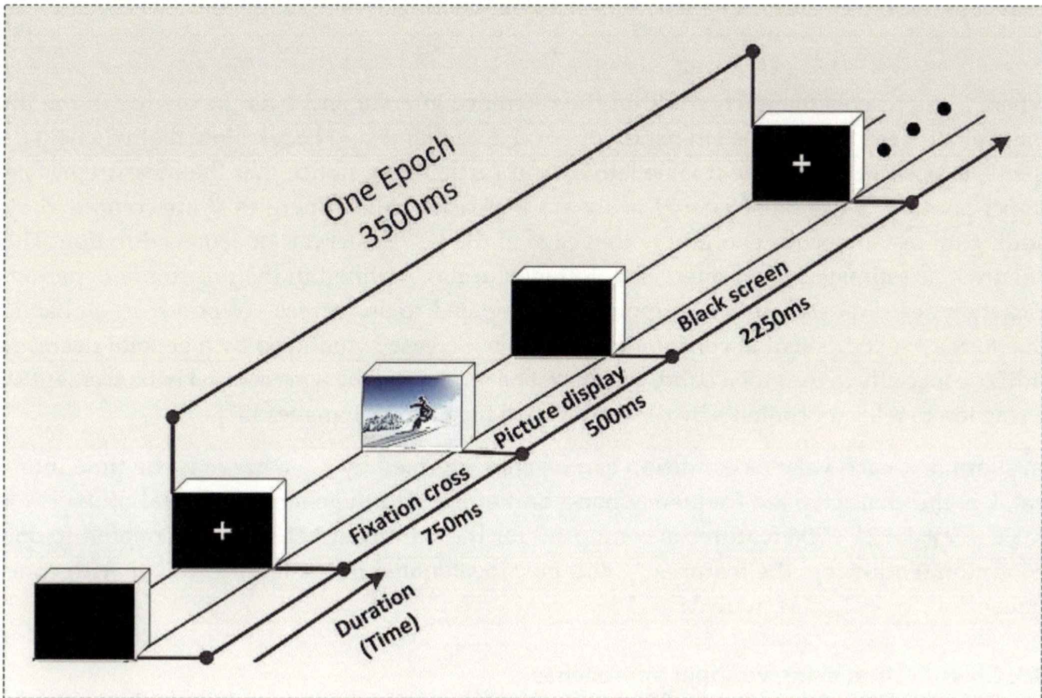

Figure 2. Experimental protocol: series of the stimuli presentation for a complete trial.

EEG activity on the scalp was recorded from 21 Ag/AgCl sintered electrodes (Fp1, Fpz, Fp2, F7, F3, Fz, F4, F8, T7, C3, Cz, C4, T8, P7, P3, Pz, P4, P8, O1, Oz, O_2) mounted on an electrode cap from EasyCap according to the international 10/20 system, internally referenced to an electrode on the tip of the nose. The impedances of all electrodes were kept below 5 kΩ. EEG signals were recorded, sampled at 1 kHz and preprocessed using software Scan 4.3. First, a notch filter centered in 50 Hz was applied to eliminate AC contribution. EEG signals were then filtered using high-pass and low-pass Butterworth filters with cutoff frequencies of 0.1 Hz and 30 Hz, respectively. The signal was baseline corrected and segmented into time-locked epochs using the stimulus onset (picture presentation) as reference. The length of the time windows was 950 ms: from 150 ms before picture onset to 800 ms after it (baseline = 1150 ms).

3.2. Feature extraction

The signals (either single trials or average segments) are filtered by four 4th-order bandpass Butterworth filters. $K = 4$ filters are applied following a zero-phase forward and reverse digital filter methodology not including any transient (see *filtfilt* MATLAB function [36]). The four frequency bands have been defined as: $\delta = Z[0.5, 4]$ Hz, $\theta = Z[4, 7]$ Hz, $\alpha = Z[8, 12]$ Hz and $\beta = Z[13, 30]$ Hz. From a technical point of view, ERD/ERS computation reduces significantly the initial sample size per trial (800 features corresponding to the time instants) to a much smaller number, optimizing the design of the classifier. For each filtered signal, the ERD/ERS is estimated in $I = 9$ intervals following the stimulus onset and with a duration of 150 ms and 50% of overlap between consecutive intervals. The reference interval corresponds to the 150 ms pre-stimulus period. For each interval, the ERD/ERS is defined as

$$f_{ik} = \frac{E_{rk} - E_{ik}}{E_{rk}} = 1 - \frac{E_{ik}}{E_{rk}} \tag{1}$$

where E_{rk} represents the energy within the reference interval and E_{ik} is the energy in the ith interval after stimulus in the kth band, for $i = 1,2,\ldots, 9$ and $k = 1,\ldots,4$. Note that when $E_{rk}>E_{ik}$, then f_{ik} is positive, otherwise it is negative. And furthermore notice that the measure has an upper bound $f_{ik} \leq 1$ because energy is always a positive value. Energies E_{ik} are computed by adding up instantaneous energies within each of the $I = 9$ intervals of 150 ms duration. The energy E_{rk} is estimated in an interval of 150 ms duration defined in the pre-stimulus period. Generally, early poststimulus components are related to an increase of power in all bands due to the evoked potential contribution and this increase is followed by a general decrease (ERD), especially in the alpha band, which can be modulated by a perceptual enhancement as a reaction to relevant contents by the presence of high arousal images [31].

In summary, each valence condition can be characterized by f_{ikc}, where i is the time interval, k is the characteristic frequency band and c refers to the channel. A total of $M = I \times K \times C = 9 \times 4 \times 21 = 756$ features is computed for the multichannel segments related to one condition. Following, the features f_{ikc} will be concatenated into a feature vector with components f_m, $m = 1,\ldots,M$, with $M = 756$.

3.3. Classification using wrapper approaches

The target of any feature selection method is the selection of the most pertinent feature subset which provides the most discriminant information from a complete feature set. In the wrapper approach, the feature selection algorithm acts as a wrapper around the classification algorithm. In this case, the feature selection consists of searching a relevant subset of features from high-dimensional data sets using the induction algorithm itself as part of the function-evaluating features [37]. Hence, the parameters of the classifier serve as scores to select (or to eliminate) features and the corresponding classification performance is the guide to an iterative procedure. The recursive feature elimination strategy using a linear SVM-based classifier is a wrapper method usually called support vector machine recursive feature elimination (SVM-RFE) [38]. This strategy was introduced when the data sets had a large number of features compared to the number of training examples [38], but it was recently applied for class-imbalanced data sets [39]. A similar strategy can be applied with other learning algorithms, for instance random-forest that has an embedded method of feature selection. The random forest is an ensemble of binary decision trees where the training is achieved by randomly selecting subsets of features. Therefore, computing a variable using parameters of the classifier, which somehow reflect the importance of each input (feature) of the classifier, an iterative procedure can be developed. Assuming that this variable importance is r_m, the steps of the wrapper method are:

1. Initialize: create a set of indices $M = \{1,2,\ldots,M\}$ relative to the available features and set $F = M$.
2. Organize data set X by forming the feature vectors with the feature values whose index is in set M, labeling each feature vector according to the class it belongs (negative or positive valence).
3. Compute the accuracy of the classifier using the leave-one-out (LOO) cross-validation strategy.
4. Compute the global model of the classifier using the complete data set X.

5. Compute r_m of the feature set and eliminate from set M the indices relative to the twenty least relevant features.

6. Update the number of features accordingly, i.e. $F \leftarrow F$ -20.

7. Repeat steps 2–6 while the number of features in set M is larger than $M_{min} = 36$.

Accuracy is the proportion of true results (either positive or negative valence) in the test set. The leave-one-out strategy assumes that only one example of the data set forms the test set while all the remaining belong to the training set. This training and test procedure is repeated so that all the elements of the data set are used once as test set (step 3 of the wrapper method). Then, after computing the model of the classifier with the complete data, the importance of each feature is estimated (steps 4 and 5).

As mentioned before, random forest and linear SVM are classifiers that can be applied in a wrapper method approach and used to estimate r_m. For convenience, the next two subsections review the relevant parameters of both classifiers and their relation to the variable importance mechanism.

3.3.1. *Random forest*

The random forest algorithm, developed by Breiman [40], is a set of binary decision trees, each performing a classification, being the final decision taken by majority voting. Each tree is grown using a bootstrap sample from the original data set and each node of the tree randomly selects a small subset of features for a split. An optimal split separates the set of samples of the node into two more homogeneous (pure) subgroups with respect to the class of its elements. A measure for the impurity level is the Gini index. By considering that ω_c, $c = 1 \ldots C$ are the labels given to the classes, the Gini index of node i is defined as

$$G(i) = 1 - \sum_{c=1}^{C} \left(P(\omega_c)\right)^2 \tag{2}$$

where $P(\omega_c)$ is the probability of class ω_c in the set of examples that belong to node i. Note that $G(i) = 0$ when node i is pure, e.g., if its data set contains only examples of one class. To perform a split, one feature f_m is tested $f_m > f_0$ on the set of samples with n elements which is then divided into two groups (left and right) with n_l and n_r elements. The change in impurity is computed as

$$\Delta G(i) = G(i) - \left(\frac{n_l}{n} G(i_l) - \frac{n_r}{n} G(i_r)\right) \tag{3}$$

The feature and value that results in the largest decrease of the Gini index is chosen to perform the split at node i. Each tree is grown independently using random feature selection to decide the splitting test of the node and no pruning is done on the grown trees. The main steps of this algorithm are

1. Given a data set T with N examples, each with F features, select the number T of trees, the dimension of the subset $L < F$ of features and the parameter that controls the size of the tree (it can be the maximum depth of the tree, the minimum size of the subset in a node to perform a split).

2. Construct the $t = 1 \ldots T$ trees.

   a. Create a training set $T\ t$ with N examples by sampling with replacement the original data set. The out-of-bag data set Ot is formed with the remaining examples of T not belonging to $T\ t$.

   b. Perform the split of node i by testing one of the $L = \sqrt{F}$ randomly selected features.

   c. Repeat step 2b until the tree t is complete. All nodes are terminal nodes (leafs) if the number n_s of examples is $n_s \leq 0.1N$.

3. Repeat step 2 to grow next tree if $t \neq T$. In this work $T = 500$ decision trees were employed.

After training, the importance r_m of each feature f_m in the ensemble of trees can be computed by adding the values of $\Delta G(i)$ of all nodes i where the feature f_m is used to perform a split. Sorting the values r by decreasing order, it is possible to identify the relative importance of the features. The $F = 20$ least relevant features are eliminated from the feature vector f.

3.3.2. Linear SVM

Linear SVM parameters define decision hyperplanes or hypersurfaces in the multidimensional feature space [41, 42], that is:

$$g(w) = w^T x + b = 0 \tag{4}$$

where $x \equiv f$ denotes the vector of features, w is known as the weight vector and b is the threshold.

The optimization task consists of finding the unknown parameters w_m, $m = 1,\ldots,F$ and b [43]. The position of the decision hyperplane is determined by vector w and b: the vector is orthogonal to the decision plane and b determines its distance to the origin. For the Linear SVM the vector w can be explicitly computed and this constitutes an advantage as it decreases the complexity during the test phase. With the optimization algorithm the Lagrangian values, $0 \leq \lambda_i \leq C$ are estimated [43]. The training examples, known as support vectors, are related with the nonzero Lagrangian coefficients. The weight vector then can be computed

$$w = \sum_{i}^{N_s} y_i \lambda_i x_i \tag{5}$$

where N_s is the number of the support vectors and (x_i, y_i) is the support vector and corresponding label {-1,1}. The threshold b is estimated as an average of the projected supported vectors $w^T x_i$ corresponding to $C \neq 0$. The value of C needs to be assigned to run the training optimization algorithm and controls the number of errors allowed versus the margin width. During the optimization process, C represents the weight of the penalty term of the optimization function that is related to the misclassification error in the training set. There is no optimal procedure to assign this parameter but it has to be expected that:

- If C is large, the misclassification errors are relevant during optimization. A narrow margin has to be expected.

- If C is small, the misclassification errors are not relevant during optimization. A large margin has to be expected.

Note that this is important because in a real application linearly separable problems are not to be expected and it is more realistic to perform an optimization where misclassifications are allowed. In the following simulations, the parameter $C = 1$ and the software MATLAB is used [44].

The relevance of the mth entry of the feature vector is then determined by the corresponding value w_m in the weight vector. In particular if $|w_m| \neq 0$, the corresponding feature do not contribute to the value of $g(w)$ [38]. Then, setting $r_m \equiv w_m$ for the SVM classifier and sorting the absolute values, the importance of the features is found out.

4. Results and discussion

To ease interpreting the following results, it is possible to link wrapper methods to some statistical contrasts (e.g. t-test) used by psychologists to test which EEG features change depending on the experimental condition. Note that in the two cases the goal is to perform a dimension reduction before the classification step. For instance, another alternative methodology would consist of transforming the initial vector of features to low-dimensional space by performing a singular value decomposition [45]. Both approaches can be considered as filter techniques to reduce the dimension of an initial feature vector. In the former, statistical analysis, the dimension reduction is achieved according to a parameter from a classifier and each feature is taken individually to check how its value influences the classification outcome. In the latter, machine learning approach, the significant features, selected from the initial vector, are obtained after comparing two sets of features belonging to two different conditions and checking a statistical value. Classification techniques have the advantage of dealing with the set of features as a whole without needing a complementary observation (belonging to another condition). Therefore, the results obtained by wrapper methods can complement the conclusions drawn by applying other statistical tests, indicating the most relevant features related to specific processes, e.g., affective valence processing.

Considering feature elimination and the concomitant number of relevant features, as can be seen from **Figures 3–6**, the accuracy of the wrapper classifiers improves with a decreasing number of relevant features in both, inter or intrasubject classification strategies. In all cases, the system achieves 80% accuracy rate using random forest whereas the system reaches values close to 100% by means of SVM when the classifier has less than 100 relevant features as input.

4.1. Intersubject classification

Figures 3 and **4** show the accuracy versus the number of removed features obtained by applying the two methods: random forest and SVM, respectively. The accuracy was computed with a LOO cross-validation strategy and a total of 52 feature vectors were involved, which represent the ensemble averages referring to positive and negative affective valence responses of all volunteers investigated (26 for each class). Each feature vector is composed of $M = 756$ elements (see section 3.2). A global accuracy of 79% is achieved by the system if roughly 500 irrelevant features are removed from the input feature set with random forest, whereas the system yields an accuracy peak value of 100% using SVM-RFE after removing 680 features, remaining less than 100 features as relevant ones.

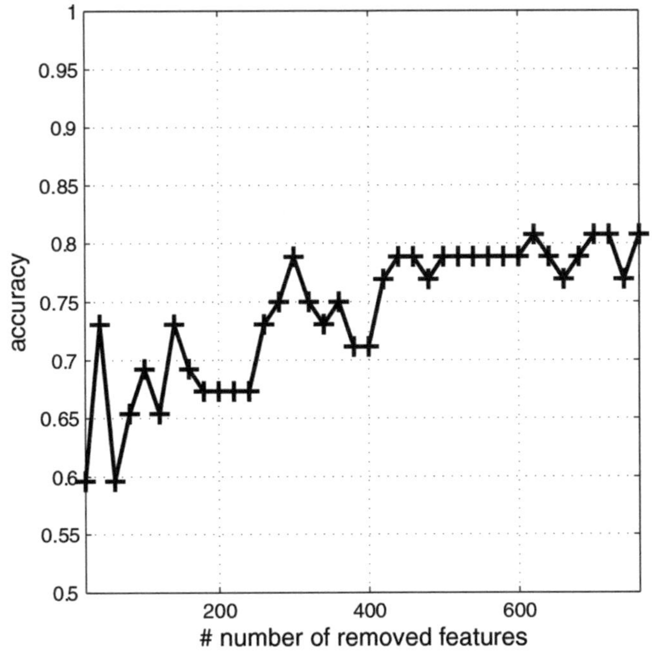

Figure 3. Intersubject accuracy obtained by the implemented random forest. Features extracted from ensemble-average signals are computed at least over 30 single trials.

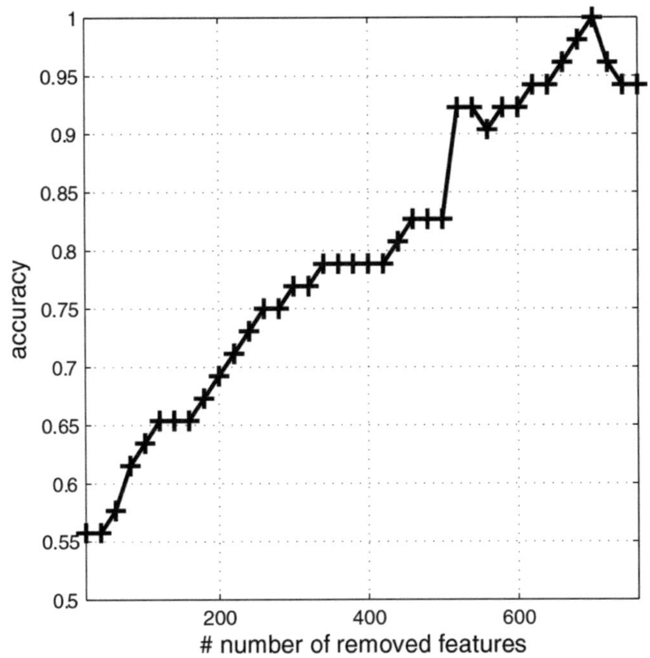

Figure 4. Intersubject accuracy obtained by the implemented SVM-RFE. Features extracted from ensemble-average signals are computed at least over 30 single trials.

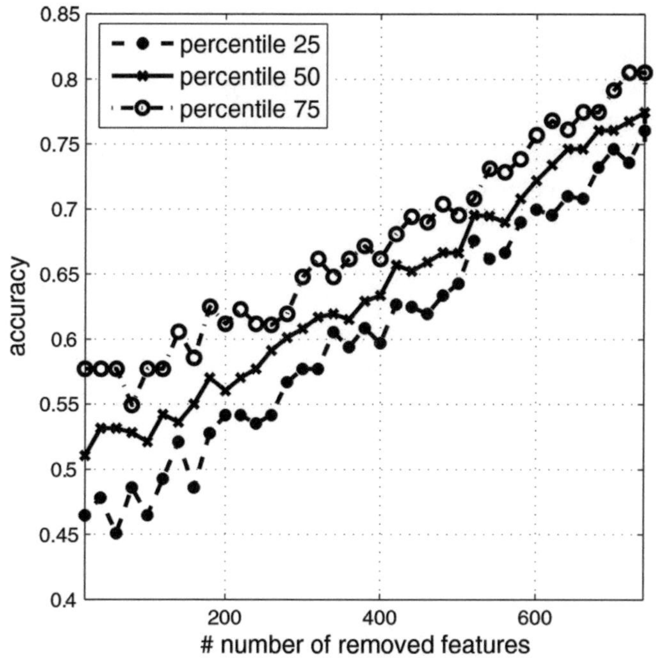

Figure 5. Intrasubject percentiles of accuracy values versus the number of features removed using random forest. The last point corresponds to 36 selected features.

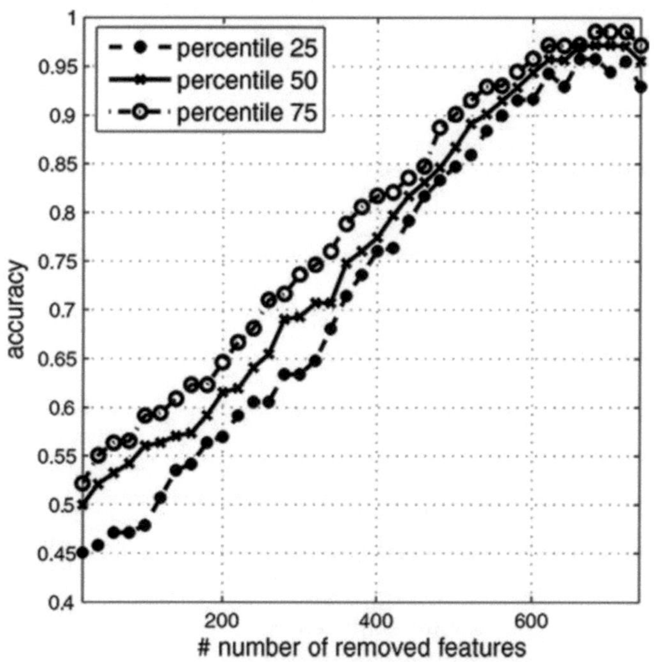

Figure 6. Intrasubject percentiles of accuracy values versus the number of features removed using SVM-RFE. The last point corresponds to 36 selected features.

Tables 1 and **2** describe the spatial and temporal locations of the relevant features when the input of the classifiers is the data set formed by these 52 feature vectors. Concerning spatial locations, both random forest and the SVM algorithm allocate the relevant features consistently in frontal regions of the brain, although SVM also keeps a significant number from centroparietal regions. This corroborates other research works where, during affective processing, the particular contribution of frontal regions has also been pointed out [46, 47]. Concerning location in time, with a random forest most of the features display *medium* and *long* latencies while with an SVM the most relevant time interval corresponds to *medium* latencies. Hence, in contrast to a random forest, the SVM selects a larger number of features from early poststimulus time intervals. These results also match previous brain studies reported in literature, in which ensembles of averaged signals were used as well [20, 48]. Note that although the two methods hardly agree to the time intervals where features show up, both highlight frontal areas as relevant spatial locations for affective valence processing.

Scalp region	Beta	Alpha	Theta	Delta	Total
Frontal	7	2	4	5	18
Central-temporal	6	0	3	0	9
Parietooccipital	5	2	0	2	9
Time interval	**Beta**	**Alpha**	**Theta**	**Delta**	**Total**
Short	0	1	0	0	1
Medium	6	1	0	2	9
Long I	12	0	1	3	16
Long II	0	2	6	2	10

Upper table: Space location (EEG channels): frontal (FP1, FPz, FP2, F7, F3, Fz, F4, F8), central-temporal (T7, C3, Cz, C4, T8) and parietal-occipital (P7, P3, Pz, P4, P8, O1, Oz, O_2). Lower table: Time location (time intervals): short (i = {1,2}), medium (i = {3.4}), long l (i = {5,6}) and long II (i = {7,8,9}).

Table 1. Distribution of the 36 selected features within each band by random forest (intersubject classification).

4.2. Intrasubject classification

Figures 5 and **6** show the global accuracy, computed by averaging the particular accuracy values of all participants, when the classifiers were trained on only one subject's data. For an intrasubject classification purpose, features were extracted from single-trial signals as described above (Section 3). The training set for each subject is made up by a total of 65-72 single trials for both classes of emotions and LOO cross-validation strategy is applied as well.

Similar to intersubject analysis, SVM-RFE yielded better results in terms of accuracy rates than random forest when features are extracted from single-trials. SVM-RFE reaches mean values close to the maximal accuracy and up to 100% for some subjects. Nevertheless, random forest keeps an 80% accuracy as the upper limit.

Scalp region	Beta	Alpha	Theta	Delta	Total
Frontal	5	6	0	5	16
Central-temporal	6	0	2	5	13
Parietooccipital	3	3	1	0	7
Time interval	**Beta**	**Alpha**	**Theta**	**Delta**	**Total**
Short	2	3	3	1	9
Medium	6	2	0	3	11
Long I	4	0	0	3	7
Long II	2	4	0	3	9

Upper table: Space location (EEG channels): frontal (Fp1, Fpz, Fp2, F7, F3, Fz, F4, F8), central-temporal (T7, C3, Cz, C4, T8) and parietal-occipital (P7, P3, Pz, P4, P8, O1, Oz, O2). Lower table: Time location (time intervals): short (i = {1,2}), medium (i = {3.4}), long l (i = {5,6}) and long II (i = {7,8,9}).

Table 2. Distribution of the 36 selected features within each band by SVM-RFE (intersubject classification).

A comparison of the outcomes of individual training sessions, with respect to the 36 features that remain, reveals a large interindividual. All training sessions encompassed an equal number of iterations. For each feature, it was then counted how often it occurred in any subject. **Figure 7** displays this comparison. It shows that, for example, 220 features never survived

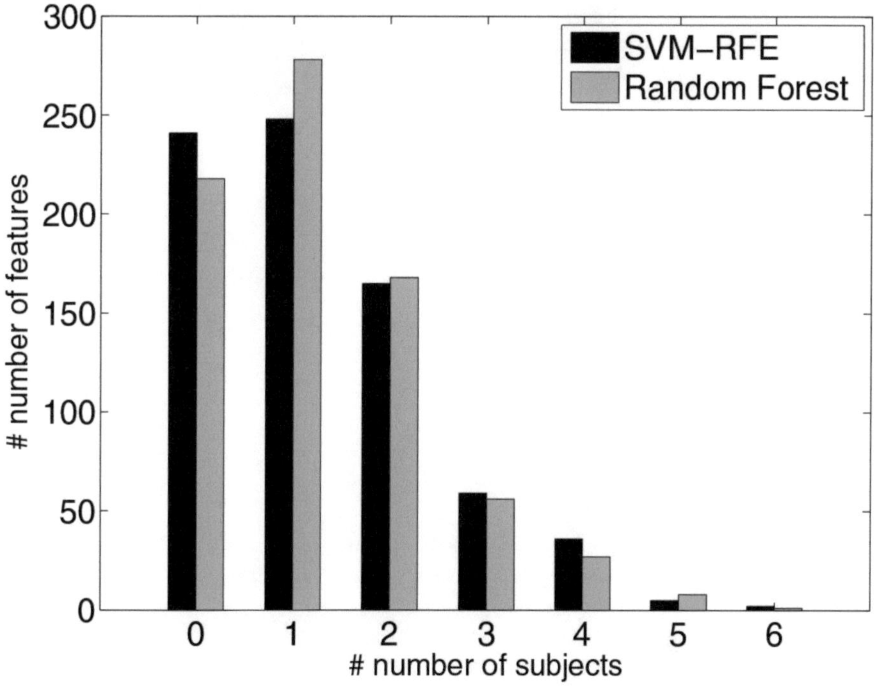

Figure 7. Within the 36 features selected from each individual training, the histogram counts the number of times a feature was selected using both wrapper methods.

in any individual thus may be considered completely irrelevant. Remarkably, few features appear consistently as relevant features in at least six out of 26 subjects confirming the high interindividual heterogeneity, independently on the applied method for selecting features. A similar conclusion was drawn in Ref. [15], in this case by using a feature selection block before performing classification. However, note that a comparable accuracy value is achieved whether decision making is based on a set of 52 feature vectors (ensemble averages over trials and subjects) or on training classifiers individually with 65–72 feature vectors for each subject.

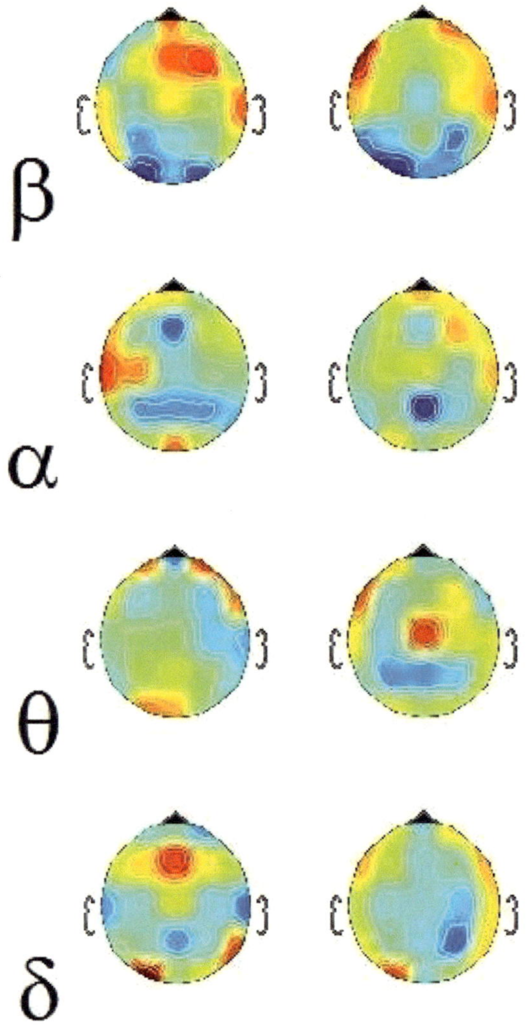

Figure 8. Spatial location of feature relevance in each frequency band obtained from counting the contribution from all subjects within intrasubject classifications (left column: random forest, right column: SVM). The relevance is represented by a color map, where blue represents the least relevant features (nonselected features) and red represents the most relevant ones (selected as relevant by all subjects).

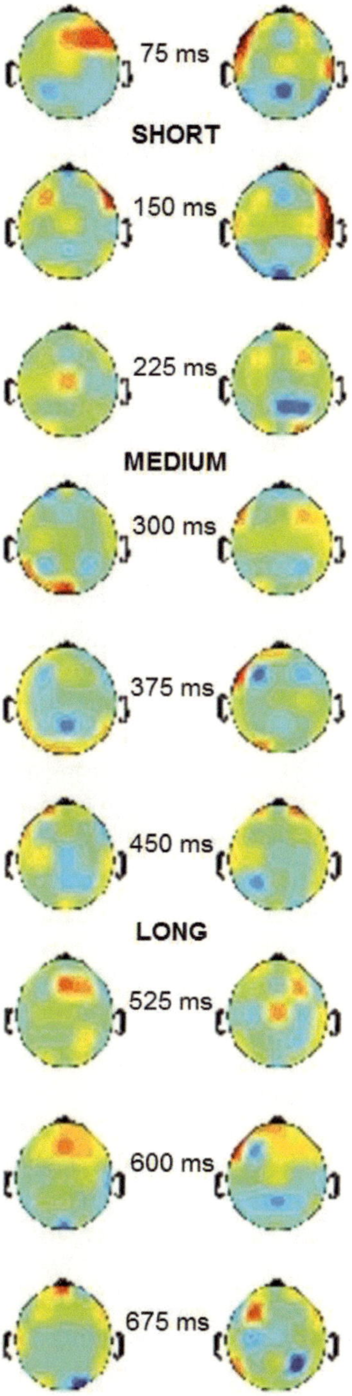

Figure 9. Relevance of the features selected for different latencies and spatial locations (left column: random forest, right column: SVM) following from counting the contribution of all subjects within an intrasubject classification. Feature importance is visualized by a normalized color map, where blue represents the least relevant features (nonselected features) and red represents the most relevant ones (selected as relevant by all subjects).

Figures 8 and **9** show the relevance of the features chosen by the two methods in topographical maps. As can be seen from **Figure 8**, on average, both algorithms allocate the most relevant features in the frontal region in agreement with intersubject applications. Similarly, both also identify relevant features mostly in the beta bands. According to **Figure 9**, both algorithms allocate important features showing up with short latencies in the frontal areas of the brain. Concerning *medium* and *long* latencies both algorithms again identify important features in frontal areas though their importance is more pronounced with the random forest.

Although intersubject and intrasubject methodologies show a similar performance, they have different application scenarios. The intersubject classification is mostly suitable for offline applications as well as for brain studies in order to complement the statistical methods. For instance, in Ref. [49], an SVM-RFE scheme was exclusively applied to identify scalp spectral dynamics linked with the affective valence processing and to compare with standard statistical results (t-test). In that work, a different technique for feature extraction was developed, whose goals consisted of creating a particular volume of features by means of a wavelet filtering. In this way, a high-dimensional data set was represented by means of three dimensions: frequency (resolution: 1 Hz), time (resolution: 1 ms) and topographical location (21 EEG channels).

Due to the biological variability observed, intrasubject studies cannot generalize easily across a cohort of subjects. Thus, intrasubject approaches might be interesting for personalized studies where subjects need to be followed up for a couple of sessions, such as in a rehabilitation therapy, or for neurofeedback-based applications. An example of an intrasubject study is reported in Ref. [50], where the neuroticism trait is analyzed using EEG to check the influence of individual differences in the emotional processing and the susceptibility of each brain region. In that work SVM was used as well, although from a different standpoint, since it was performed in subject identification tasks from single trials.

5. Conclusions

A novel valence recognition system has been presented and applied to EEG signals, which were recorded from volunteers subjected to emotional states elicited by pictures drawn from IAPS repository. A cohort of 26 female participants has been investigated. The recognition system encompasses a feature extraction stage and a classification module including feature elimination. The complete system focused on both an intersubject and an intrasubject situation. Both studies show a similar performance with regard to the classification accuracy. The recursive feature elimination (selection) was designed based on a random forest classifier or support vector machine and increased the initial classification accuracy in a range from 20% to 45%. The importance measures from both algorithms point to frontal areas although no consistent set of features and related latencies could be identified.

This fact points toward a large biological variability of the set of relevant features corresponding to the valence of the emotional states involved. In any case, the classification accuracy achieved compares well with or is even superior to competing systems reported in the literature.

http://dx.doi.org/10.5772/66667

Comparing both classifiers, the SVM achieves better classification accuracy, yielding up to 100% accuracy rate for several subjects by using the selected features for intrasubject classification task, outperforming random forest that reached an 81% maximum peak accuracy. Furthermore, the presented wrapper methods are a good option to greatly reduce the dimension of the input space and deserve to be considered as an alternative for discriminating relevant scalp regions, frequency bands and time intervals from EEG recordings.

Author details

Antonio R. Hidalgo-Muñoz[1*], Míriam M. López[1], Isabel M. Santos[2], Manuel Vázquez-Marrufo[3], Elmar W. Lang[4] and Ana M. Tomé[1]

*Address all correspondence to: arhidalgom@gmail.com

1 IEETA, University of Aveiro, Aveiro, Portugal

2 CITENSIS, Department of Education and Psychology, University of Aveiro, Aveiro, Portugal

3 University of Seville, Seville, Spain

4 Biophysics CIML Group, University of Regensburg, Regensburg, Germany

References

[1] S. A. Calvo, S. D'Mello. Affect detection: an interdisciplinary review of models, methods and their applications. IEEE Transactions on Affective Computing. 2010;**1**(1):18–37.

[2] J. L. Salmerón. Fuzzy cognitive maps for artificial emotions forecasting. Applied Soft Computing. 2012;**12**:3704–3710.

[3] M. Krauledat, K. Grzeska, M. Sagebaum, B. Blankertz, C. Vidaurre, K. R. Mïller, M. Schrïder. Playing pinball with non-invasive BCI. In: Advances in Neural Information Processing Systems 21; 2009. pp. 1641–1648. Edited by D. Koller and D. Schuurmans and Y. Bengio and L. Bottou Publisher: Curran Associates, Inc. New York (USA).

[4] D. Huang, K. Qian, D. Fei, W. Jia, X. Chen, O. Bai. Electroencephalography (EEG)-based brain-computer interface (BCI): A 2-D virtual wheelchair control based on event-related desynchronization/synchronization and state control. IEEE transactions on Neural Systems and Rehabilitation engineering. 2012;**20**(3):379–388.

[5] J. A. Russell. A circumplex model of affect. Journal of Personality and Social Psychology. 1980;**39**(6):1161–1178.

[6] M. M. Bradley, P. J. Lang. The international affective picture system (IAPS) in the study of emotion and attention. In: M. M. Bradley, P. J. Lang, editors. Handbook of Emotion Elicitation and Assessment. Oxford University Press; Oxford. 2007. pp. 29–46.

[7] C. Mühl, B. Allison, A. Nijholt, G. Chanel. A survey of affective brain computer interfaces: principles, state-of-the-art and challenges. Brain-Computer Interfaces. 2014;**1**(2):62–84.

[8] J. Klein, Y. Moon, R. W. Picard. This computer responds to user frustration: theory, design and results. Interacting with Computers. 2002;**14**(2):119–140.

[9] P. Lang, M. Bradley, B. Cuthbert. International affective picture system (IAPS): Affective ratings of pictures and instruction manual. Technical Report. 2008.

[10] S. Koelstra, C. Muhl, M. Soleymani, J.-S. Lee, A. Yazdani, T. Ebrahimi, T. Pun, A. Nijholt, I. Patras. DEAP: a database for emotion analysis; using physiological signals. IEEE Transactions on Affective Computing. 2012;**3**(1):18–31.

[11] R. W. Picard, E. Vyzas, J. Healey. Toward machine emotional intelligence: analysis of affective physiological state. IEEE Transactions on Pattern Analysis and Machine Intelligence. 2001;**23**(10):1175–1191.

[12] A. Haag, S. Goronzy, P. Schaich, J. Williams. Emotion recognition using bio-sensors: First steps towards an automatic system. In: E. André, L. Dybkjær, W. Minker, P. Heisterkamp, editors. Affective Dialogue Systems. 6th ed. Springer Berlin Heidelberg; Berlin. 2004. pp. 36–48.

[13] K. H. Kim, S. W. Bang, S. R. Kim. Emotion recognition system using short-term monitoring of physiological signals. Medical & Biological Engineering & Computing. 2004;**42**(3):419–427.

[14] K. Schaaff, T. Schultz. Towards emotion recognition from electroencephalographic signals. In: IEEE, editor. 3rd International Conference on Affective Computing and Intelligent Interaction and Workshops (ACII), 2009; 2009. pp. 1–6. (sede física de IEEE: New York).

[15] M. Macas, M. Vavrecka, V. Gerla, L. Lhotska. Classification of the emotional states based on the EEG signal processing. In: IEEE, editor. 9th International Conference on Information Technology and Applications in Biomedicine; November 2009; 2009. pp. 1–4. New York.

[16] C. A. Frantzidis, C. Bratsas, M. A. Klados, E. Konstantinidis, C. D. Lithari, A. B. Vivas, C. L. Papadelis, E. Kaldoudi, C. Pappas, P. D. Bamidis. On the classification of emotional biosignals evoked while viewing affective pictures: An integrated data-mining-based approach for healthcare applications. IEEE Transactions on Information Technology in Biomedicine. 2010;**14**(2):309–318.

[17] P. Petrantonakis, L. Hadjileontiadis. Emotion recognition from brain signals using hybrid adaptive filtering and higher order crossings analysis. IEEE Transactions on Affective Computing. 2010;**1**(2):81–97.

[18] P. C. Petrantonakis, L. J. Hadjileontiadis. Emotion recognition from EEG using higher order crossings. IEEE Transactions on Information Technology in Biomedicine. 2010;**14**(2):186–197.

[19] Q. Zhang, M. Lee. Emotion development system by interacting with human EEG and natural scene understanding. Cognitive Systems Research. 2012;**14**(1):37–49.

[20] J. K. Olofsson, S. Nordin, H. Sequeira, J. Polich. Affective picture processing: an integrative review of ERP findings. Biological Psychology. 2008;**77**(3):247–265.

[21] C. Lithari, C. Frantzidis, C. Papadelis, A. B. Vivas, M. Klados, C. Kourtidou-Papadeli, C. Pappas, A. Ioannides, P. Bamidis. Are females more responsive to emotional stimuli? A neurophysiological study across arousal and valence dimensions. Brain Topography. 2010;**23**(1):27–40.

[22] X. J. Wang. Neurophysiological and computational principles of cortical rhythms in cognition. Physiological Reviews. 2010;**90**(3):1195–1268.

[23] W. J. Ray, H. W. Cole. EEG alpha activity reflects attentional demands and beta activity reflects emotional and cognitive processes. Science. 1985;**228**(4700):750–752.

[24] E. Beraha, J. Eggers, C. H. Attar, S. Gutwinski, F. Schlagenhauf, M. Stoy, P. Sterzer, T. Kienast, A. Heinz, F. Bermpohl. Hemispheric asymmetry for affective stimulus processing in healthy subjects – a fMRI study. PLoS One. 2012;**7**(10):e46931.

[25] H. J. Yoon, S. Y. Chung. EEG spectral analysis in valence and arousal dimensions of emotion. In: 11th International Conference on Control, Automation and Systems (ICCAS); October 2011. pp. 1319–1322 IEEE.

[26] G. Pfurtscheller, F. H. Lopes da Silva. Event-related EEG/MEG synchronization and desynchronization: basic principles. Clinical Neurophysiology. 1999;**110** (11):1842–1857.

[27] L. Aftanas, A. Varlamow, S. Pavlov, V. Makhnev, N. Reva. Affective picture processing: event-related synchronization within individually defined human theta band is modulated by valence dimension. Neuroscience Letters. 2001;**303**(2):115–118.

[28] L. I. Aftanas, N. V. Reva, A. A. Varlamov, S. V. Pavlov, V. P. Makhnev. Analysis of evoked EEG synchronization and desynchronization in conditions of emotional activation in humans: temporal and topographic characteristics. Neuroscience and Behavioral Physiology. 2004;**34**(8):859–867.

[29] G. Knyazev, J. Slobodskoj-Plusnin, A. Bocharov. Event-related delta and theta synchronization during explicit and implicit emotion processing. Neuroscience. 2009;**164**(4):1588–1600.

[30] M. A. Klados, C. Frantzidis, A. B. Vivas, C. Papadelis, C. Lithari, C. Pappas, P. D. Bamidis. A framework combining delta event-related oscillations (EROs) and synchronisation effects (ERD/ERS) to study emotional processing. In: Computational Intelligence and Neuroscience; The ACM Digital Library. January; 2009. p. 12.

[31] A. De Cesarei, M. Codispoti. Affective modulation of the LPP and alpha-ERD during picture viewing. Psychophysiology. 2011;**48**(10):1397–1404.

[32] A. Delorme, S. Makeig. EEGLAB: an open source toolbox for analysis of single-trial EEG dynamics including independent component analysis. Journal of Neuroscience Methods. 2004;**134**(1):9–21.

[33] A. Jaiantilal, http://code.google.com/p/randomforest-matlab/, 2010.

[34] A. H. Kemp, R. B. Silberstein, S. M. Armstrong, P. J. Nathan. Gender differences in the cortical electrophysiological processing of visual emotional stimuli. Neuroimage. 2004; **21**(2):632–646.

[35] K. Schaaff. Challenges on emotion induction with the international affective picture system. 2008. [Online]. Available: http://csl.ira. uka.de/fileadmin/media/publication files/ SA-Schaaff.pdf

[36] Mathworks, 2012. [Online]. Available: http://www.mathworks.com/help/signal/ref/filtfilt.html

[37] R. Kohavi and G. H. John. Wrappers for feature subset selection. Artificial Intelligence. 1997;**97**(1–2):273–324.

[38] I. Guyon, J. Weston, S. Barnhill, V. Vapnik. Gene selection for cancer classification using support vector machines. Machine Learning. 2002;**46**(1–3):389–422.

[39] S. Maldonado, R. Weber, F. Famili. Feature selection for high-dimensional class-imbalanced data sets using support vector machines. Information Sciences. 2014;**286**(0):228–246. [Online]. Available: http://www.sciencedirect.com/science/article/pii/S0020025514007154

[40] L. Breiman. Random forests. Machine Learning. 2001;**45**(2): 5–32.

[41] C. J. C. Burges. A tutorial on support vector machines for pattern recognition. Data Mining and Knowledge Discovery. 1998;**2**(2):121–167.

[42] I. A. Illan, J. M. Gorriz, M. M. Lopez, J. Ramirez, D. Salas-Gonzalez, F. Segovia, R. Chaves, C. G. Puntonet. Computer aided diagnosis of Alzheimer's disease using component based SVM. Applied Soft Computing. 2011;**11**(2):2376–2382.

[43] A. Ben-Hur, C. Ong, S. Sonnenburg, B. Schölkopf, G. Rätsch. Support vector machines and kernels for computational biology. PLoS Computational Biology. 2008;**10**(4):e1000173.

[44] Bioinformatics-Toolbox, 2012. [Online]. Available: http://www. mathworks.com

[45] S. N. Daimi, G. Saha. Classification of emotions induced by music videos and correlation with participants rating. Expert Systems with Applications. 2014;**41**(13):6057–6065. [Online]. Available: http://www.sciencedirect.com/science/article/pii/S0957417414001882

[46] R. J. Davidson, W. Irwin. The functional neuroanatomy of emotion and affective style. Trends in Cognitive Sciences. 1999;**3**(1):11–21.

[47] S. K. Sutton, R. J. Davidson. Prefrontal brain electrical asymmetry predicts the evaluation of affective stimuli. Neuropsychologia. 2000;**38**(13):1723–1733.

[48] L. R. R. Gianotti, P. L. Faber, M. Schuler, R. D. Pascual-Marqui, K. Kochi, D. Lehmann. First valence, then arousal: the temporal dynamics of brain electric activity evoked by emotional stimuli. Brain Topography. 2008;**20**(3):143–156.

[49] A. R. Hidalgo-Muñoz, M. M. Lopez, I. M. Santos, A. T. Pereira, M. Vazquez-Marrufo, A. Galvao-Carmona, A. M. Tome. Application of SVM-RFE on EEG signals for detecting the most relevant scalp regions linked to affective valence processing. Expert Systems with Applications. 2013;**40**(6):2102–2108.

[50] A. R. Hidalgo-Muñoz, A. T. Pereira, M. M. Lopez, A. Galvao-Carmona, A. M. Tome, M. Vazquez-Marrufo, I. M. Santos. Individual EEG differences in affective valence processing in women with low and high neuroticism. Clinical Neurophysiology. 2013;**124**(9):1798–1806.

Chapter 4

Tracking the Sound of Human Affection: EEG Signals Reveal Online Decoding of Socio-Emotional Expression in Human Speech and Voice

Xiaoming Jiang

Additional information is available at the end of the chapter

http://dx.doi.org/10.5772/66418

Abstract

This chapter provides a perspective from the latest EEG evidence in how brain signals enlighten the neurophysiological and neurocognitive mechanisms underlying the recognition of socioemotional expression conveyed in human speech and voice, drawing upon event-related potentials' studies (ERPs). Human sound can encode emotional meanings by different vocal parameters in words, real- vs. pseudo-speeches, and vocalizations. Based on the ERP findings, recent development of the three-stage model in vocal processing has highlighted initial- and late-stage processing of vocal emotional stimuli. These processes, depending on which ERP components they were mapped onto, can be divided into the acoustic analysis, relevance and motivational processing, fine-grained meaning analysis/integration/access, and higher-level social inference, as the unfolding of the time scale. ERP studies on vocal socioemotions, such as happiness, anger, fear, sadness, neutral, sincerity, confidence, and sarcasm in the human voice and speech have employed different experimental paradigms such as crosssplicing, crossmodality priming, oddball, stroop, etc. Moreover, task demand and listener characteristics affect the neural responses underlying the decoding processes, revealing the role of attention deployment and interpersonal sensitivity in the neural decoding of vocal emotional stimuli. Cultural orientation affects our ability to decode emotional meaning in the voice. Neurophysiological patterns were compared between normal and abnormal emotional processing in the vocal expressions, especially in schizophrenia and in congenital amusia. Future directions highlight the study on human vocal expression aligning with other nonverbal cues, such as facial and body language, and the need to synchronize listener's brain potentials with other peripheral measures.

Keywords: affective voice, social communication, nonverbal cues, pragmatics, EEG/ERPs, empathy, anxiety, person perception

1. Introduction

Theoretical models based on electrophysiological studies have indicated early and late neurophysiological markers that index online perception of vocal emotion expressions in speech as well as other higher-order socioemotive expressions (e.g., confidence, sarcasm, sincerity, etc.), which roughly correspond to each hypothesized processing stage [1, 2]. Studies with event-related potentials (ERPs), which focused on the analysis of averaged electrophysiological response to a certain vocal or speech event, have enlightened neurocognitive processes at a fine-grained temporal scale. The early fronto-central auditory N1 is known to be associated with a wide range of auditory stimulus types as a measure of sensory-perceptual processing. In vocal emotion processing, N1 has been linked to the extraction of acoustic cues that differentiate different types of vocal signals, frequency, and intensity parameters [3, 4], and is unaffected by differences in emotional meaning. The fronto-central P200 has been associated with the early attentional allocation or relevance evaluation of vocal signals [2, 5], ensuring preferential processing of emotional stimuli. Differentiation of P200 amplitude can be found between basic emotions [6] or between emotional vs. neutral speech [3, 7], suggesting that this component may reflect an early function of "tagging" emotional or motivational relevant stimuli. The P200 tended to be associated with higher mean and range of f0, larger mean and range of amplitude of speech, and slower speech rate [6], implicating that the early P200 modulation is partially explained by early meaning encoding as well as continued sensory processing [8]. A late centro-parietal positivity (also named LPC) evoked by vocal emotion expressions has been defined as a positive-going wave starting about 500 ms post-onset of the vocal stimuli and perhaps sustaining until 1200 ms depending on stimulus features. The LPC is considered as reflecting continued or second-pass evaluative process of the meaning of vocal emotional signals [2, 5]. The LPC was larger in emotional vocal stimuli, leading to larger differences in the LPC amplitude among basic emotion types [6], suggesting a more elaborative processing vocal information at this stage. In addition to these ERP effects, a more delayed sustained positivity may reflect a listener's attempt to infer the goal of a speaker, especially when an expected way of speaking is mismatched in an utterance context [9]. These event-related potential components have provided a useful tool to examine the temporal neural dynamics of emotional decoding in voice and speech.

2. Neurophysiological studies on basic vocal emotion in speech and voice

Vocal emotion has been investigated mainly in vocalization and speech. A study compared the ERP responses toward the perception of three basic emotions (happiness, sadness, and anger) in vocalization vs. pseudo-speech (same as real-speech except the lexical-semantic contents were replaced by meaningless syllables [10, 11]) in a task when listeners were presented with emotional vocal expressions followed by emotional and neutral faces and were asked to judge the emotionality of the face. Pell et al. [11] showed that the vocalization and speech can be differentiated very early at about 100 ms. Vocalization elicited a larger, earlier, and more differentiated P200 between emotions, and a stronger and earlier late-positivity effect. These findings support a preferential decoding in the neurophysiological system of vocalization over speech-embedded emotions in the human voice. They also demonstrated angry voice elicited the strongest P200 than the other expressions. In another study in which anger, happiness, and neutral vocalizations were compared, anger elicited a stronger positivity in the 50 ms while both anger and happiness elicited a reduced N100 and an increased P200 as compared with neutral vocalization [7]. These findings, taken together, suggest an early sensory registration of emotional information which is assigned increased relevance or motivational significance in decoding human vocalization.

Earlier ERP works have focused on how the brain responded to emotional transitions in the voice and to the transition in both voice and lexico-semantics simultaneously [13]. Using a crosssplicing technique, a leading phrase of a sentence was crossspliced with the main stem of a sentence either congruent or incongruent in prosody with the leading phrase. The onset of the crosssplicing point of the vocal expression in the main sentence elicited a larger negativity (350–550 ms) for a mismatch in both voice and lexico-semantics and a larger more right-hemispheric distributed positivity (600–950 ms) for a mismatch in voice only (pseudo-utterances: [3]; utterances with no emotional lexical items: [1]). The negativity suggested an effort of integrating the emotional information in both vocal and semantic channel with the context. The late positivity suggests a detection of acoustic variation in the vocal expression.

Some evidence further delineated the role of a specific acoustic feature in the ERP responses toward the vocal emotion decoding. For example, one EEG study compared the ERPs for the mismatching emotional prosody (a statement with neutral voice which was disrupted by an anger voice) and that for the matching prosody revealed an increased N2/P3 as compared with the matching prosody ([12]). The amplitude of the N2/P3 complex was reduced and the latency of such complex was more delayed when the intensity for that prosody was weakened. This finding suggests that emotional significance in the voice can be promoted by increased sound intensity. The role of a specific acoustic profile such as loudness of sound needs to be specified in vocal-emotion studies.

3. Neurophysiological studies on vocal sarcasm, sincerity and confidence

In order to evaluate whether and how basic emotional and higher-level social information (e.g., attitudinal) are manifested in the brain in a different manner, Wickens and Perry [13] compared the ERP responses to neutral, angry, and sarcastic expressions. These expressions began with a leading phrase (e.g., He has) in a neutral voice and were followed by an expression (e.g., a serious face) intoned with different voices. As compared with the neutral expression, both angry and sarcastic expression elicited an increased P200 and a late positivity effect (450–700 ms) with no amplitude difference between the two emotions. The angry voice also elicited an early N100 as compared with the other two expressions when listeners performed a probe-verification task. These findings revealed similar neurocognitive processes between basic emotion and interpersonal attitudes conveyed in the voice while the basic emotion seems to be registered earlier under certain conditions. Other studies revealed that the decoding of sarcasm involved similar neurocognitive processes to social intention perception. Rigoulot et al. [14] compared compliments with sincere vs. insincere tone of voice (What do you think of my presentation? I think it is very interesting) and found that the sincere compliment to the question elicited a larger P600 effect as compared with the insincere one. This ERP effect was localized in the left insula which is associated with the action of lying and concealment.

Recent growing evidence has been accumulated in the field of decoding of speaker's feeling of (un)knowing using event-related potentials. In Jiang and Pell [15], vocal expression of confidence was manipulated such that statements which sounded very confident, somewhat confident, and unconfident and those which sounded neutral were presented to native English speakers. At the onset of the vocal expression, the confident expression elicited an increased positive response than the other two types of expressions. The unconfident expression elicited an increased P300 as compared with the confident and the neutral expression. The neutral voice produced a more-delayed positivity as compared with all confidence-intending expressions.

Two follow-up experiments further evaluated how the decoding of vocal confidence expression is impacted by the presence of additional linguistic cues which either congruent [16] or incongruent [17] with the tone of voice in statements which followed the linguistic cues. Different from the statements with no lexical cues, statements with congruent cues (e.g., I'm sure; Maybe) elicited an increased N1 and P2 for confident than for unconfident and close-to-confident expressions, and an enhanced delayed positivity in unconfident and close-to-confident expression than confident one. Moreover, the direct comparison between statements with and without a preceding lexical phrase elicited a reduced N1, P2, and N400 in those without a phrase [16]. The incongruent cues elicited different ERP effects at the onset of the main statement of confident and unconfident tones. The unconfident statement elicited an increased N400 or late positivity (depending on the listener's gender). The confident statement elicited a more delayed, sustained positivity effect. Source localization of these ERP effects revealed pre-SMA for N400, suggesting a difficulty in accessing the speaker meaning, and SFG, STG and insula underlying the late positivity effect, suggesting an increased demand of executive control to implement the attentional resources and socioevaluative processes [17]. These studies extended the neurocognitive model for basic vocal emotion and argued for a perspective of studying the neurophysiological mechanisms underlying decoding interpersonal and sociointeractive affective voice.

4. Modulation of brain responses toward vocal expression by other nonverbal expressions

One of the key questions in emotional communication is how decoding vocal information is aided by other nonverbal cues. The neurophysiological studies have focused on emotional processing when voice is paired with other nonverbal social cues (such as face). In a task when participants were asked to evaluate the actor's identity (e.g., monkey or not) rather than the emotion, the simultaneous presentation of vocal and facial expressions revealed some similar ERP correlates of emotional information as the vocal expression did [18]. The bimodal emotional cues elicited a larger P200 and P300 for happy and angry expressions and a larger N250 for neutral expression, suggesting that an implicit affective processing of audiovisual information emerges as early as 200 ms. Using a priming paradigm in which a face was followed by a vocal expression of words either congruent or incongruent with the emotion of the facial expression (happiness vs. anger), Diamond and Zhang [19] revealed that the mismatch elicited an increased N400 followed by a late positivity. Further, source localization of these two effects revealed activations in the superior temporal gyrus and inferior parietal gyrus dominated in the right hemisphere.

The interaction between vocal and other nonverbal emotional information was also examined in detection of emotional change. In a study in which participants were presented with simultaneously presented vocal and facial expressions while being asked to detect the change of emotion from neutral to anger or happiness conveyed in voice or in face [20]. The P3 associated with the detection of the emotional categorical change in both voice and face was larger than the sum of the change in single channel (see also [21]). The N1 associated with the detection of early acoustic change was dependent on whether their attention was guided to the voice or the face, with the attention to the voice yielding to a N1 in bimodal change larger than the sum of the two single modal change conditions. These findings suggest the modulation of selection attention on voice-face integration during emotional change perception in early sensory processing.

5. Effects of task demand, listener characteristics, and speaker characteristics on brain responses toward vocal expression decoding

Decoding emotion from voice has suffered from many variations, one noticeable factor is the communication context. The task relevance modulates the level of explicitness of emotional processing of vocal expression. One study presented mismatching and matching emotional prosody to listeners and asked them to judge the emotional congruency (where the emotional information is task relevant), or to verify the consistency between a visually presented lexical item and the statement [22]. Three ERP effects were elicited: an early negativity effect from 150 to 250 ms regardless of task relevance and the pattern of mismatch, an early positivity from 250 to 450 ms only on angry voice which was preceded by a neutral voice but regardless task relevance, and a late positivity effect after 450 ms for the task that directed listener's attention to the emotional aspects of the vocal expression. Explicit task relevant processing emotionality enhanced vigilance in perceiving emotional change in the voice.

Vocal emotion decoding is also characterized according to the listener's characteristics. Developmental studies revealed neurophysiological correlates of emotional voice processing (especially negative emotion) were similar in children and adults [23]. Using emotional interjections ("ah"), Chronaki et al. [23] compared angry, happy, and neutral voices in 6- to 11-year-old typically developing children. The N400 was attenuated by angry than by other expression types over parietal and occipital regions. Comparing neurocognitive processes along stages of early human development merits further examinations [24].

Another topic is how listener's linguistic and cultural background affect their perception of vocal expressions. In a recent EEG study, native North-American English and Chinese speakers were asked to detect the emotion of the vocal or facial expression in a voice-face pair [25]. The emotional information between the voice and face was either congruent or incongruent. Both groups were sensitive to the emotional differences between voice and face, revealing lower accuracy and higher N400 amplitude for the incongruent voice-face pairs. However, English speakers showed more pronounced N400 enlargement and more reduced accuracy when vocal information was attended, suggesting that those from a Western culture suffered from a larger interference effect from irrelevant face information. Another study using a passive odd-ball paradigm in which the two groups of listeners were presented with deviant or standard facial expressions which were paired with a vocal expression or not [26]. Chinese speakers showed a larger mismatch negativity when vocal expression was presented together with a facial expression, suggesting that individuals from an eastern culture were more sensitive to an interference from task-irrelevant vocal cues. These findings implicate a role of cultural learning and different cultural practices in communication shape neurocognitive processes associated with the early perception of voice-face emotional cues.

Listener's biological sex has been central in modulating the integration of emotional information in vocal and verbal channels [27, 28]. Recent evidence extended this idea beyond the basic emotion. Jiang and Pell [15] examined the sex difference in evaluating confidence in both confidence- and neutral-intending vocal expressions and the associated neural responses. They revealed that the delayed positivity effect elicited by neutral-intending expression was only observed in female listeners, suggesting an inferential process aimed at deriving speaker meaning from nonexpression-intending vocal expressions. Their further analysis revealed that, when vocal statements were led by lexical phrases of some level of certainty (LEX + VOC), females elicited more pronounced N1 in confident expression and larger late positivity (550–1200 ms) in unconfident and close-to-confident expressions. When these statements were compared with those with only vocal cues signifying confidence (VOC only), reduced N1, P2 as well as N400 were observed in females [16]. These findings suggest the enhanced sensitivity to socioemotional information for females in vocal communication. Females and males also engage different strategies in resolving conflicting information in vocal expressions. Jiang and Pell [17] demonstrated that the conflicting message of vocal confidence expressions elicited different ERP effects in female vs. male listeners. The confident statement following an unconfident phrase elicited a larger delayed positivity only in a female participant; while the unconfident statement following a confident phrase elicited an N400 in a male participant and a P600 effect in male participants. These findings provided a picture of how mixed messages are dealt with in female vs. male brain: in face of a mismatch in vocal expressions, the female attempted to unify separate information to establish an integrated representation while the male updated the initially built representation by switching an alternative interpretation (for example, by saying "She has access to the building" in the unconfident voice following "I'm certain," the speaker reveals some level of hesitation).

Given its sociointeractive nature, inferring a speaker meaning from interactive emotive expression is susceptible to listener's traits and personality characteristics. One factor which has been ignored but should be evaluated is the individual's interpersonal sensitivity. Jiang and Pell [16, 17] measured individual's interpersonal sensitivity using interpersonal reactivity index (IRI) [29] and regressed the early and late ERP responses toward perceiving a certain level of confidence to the interpersonal sensitivity. They found that those who displayed higher IRI score revealed more pronounced delayed positivity effects in close-to-confident and unconfident congruent expressions [16] and in incongruent confident expressions preceded by an unconfident phrase [17]. A further examination of such individual difference revealed that a larger positivity for a female listener fully mediated their perceptual adjustment toward that incongruent expression (e.g., judging the incongruent confident expression to be less confident than the congruent one).

Listener's level of anxiety also places an important role in modulating their neural responses toward decoding vocal emotions. In Jiang and Pell [15], both early (N100) and late ERP responses (P200, late positivity) were associated with the one's trait anxiety with those exhibiting higher trait anxiety revealed a reduced N100 and late positive effect in both vocalization and speech but an enhanced P200 effect in vocalization. Jiang and Pell [17] further found that the P200 in response to the confident vs. unconfident vocal expression was larger in those who displayed a lower level of trait anxiety and such modulation mediated the reduced P200 in male listeners who showed reduced anxiety as compared with female listeners.

6. Brain responses toward vocal expression in clinical populations

The study on vocal emotion decoding in normal populations has provided a wide range of neurophysiological markers and experimental paradigms to examine how such process is impaired in a clinical context. Studies have been focusing on psychiatric-risk populations and neurodevelopment disorders.

A study used an oddball paradigm in which a group of healthy listeners with anxious and depressive tendencies and a group of controls detected the target of emotional stimuli from a sequence of neutral expressions [30]. The emotional expressions were presented in voice, in face, or in voice-face pair with congruent expressions. The amplitude of P3b in response to the deviant expression was reduced in the clinical group than the control group, only in voice-face presentation. This finding suggests the crossmodal design as an effective approach to increase the sensitivity of the P300 amplitude difference between healthy populations and those with clinical symptoms.

Another study used an auditory oddball paradigm in which anger or happy deviant vocal or nonvocal synthesized syllables (data) were presented in a sequence of neutral syllables to listeners with symptoms in schizophrenia and normal listeners [31]. A larger mismatch of negativity was elicited following the deviant angry voice and anger-bearing nonvocal sounds and such enlargement was decreased in those with schizophrenia. The weaker the MMN amplitudes, the more positive symptoms of schizophrenia. Using MMN responses to anger voice, anger-derived nonvocal sound could predict whether someone received a clinical diagnosis of schizophrenia. These findings implicate that the emotional salience detection of voices differentiate the negative and positive symptoms in neuropsychiatric disorders at the preattentive level.

The emotional prosody was also examined in those with congenital amusia (a specific neurodevelopmental disorder featured as tone-deafness, [32]). Lu et al. [32] presented emotional words spoken with declarative or the question voice to the amusics and their healthy control. The N1 was reduced and the N2 was increased in incongruent voice. The modulation of N1 was intact whereas the change in N2 was reduced in amusics, suggesting an impaired conflict processing in amusia. The authors argued that the impaired discrimination of speech intonation among amusic individuals may arise from an inability to access information extracted at early processing stages.

7. Applications and future directions

One application of these studies is to build an artificial intelligence to decode brain signals which contribute to socioemotion understanding. Most of the studies use the acted (posted) vocal expression as testing materials, which were produced by professional actors, public speakers, or amateurs to portray an intended emotion. In real-life communication, the communicators may use such emotional pose to achieve certain communicative goals. Some research purpose, for example, the cultural display in vocal expression communication, may be specifically favored by using posed stimuli. However, a call for research on naturalistic, ecological, and observation-based stimuli is highly recommended. Therefore, a future study is to examine how the brain differentiates "real" vs. "fake" vocal expression by looking at the neurophysiological responses.

Another implication of using EEG signals to study vocal emotion decoding is to test the effectiveness of speech-coding strategies used in hearing aids for deaf listeners when they distinguish the emotions via prosody-specific features of language [33, 34]. In Agrawal et al. [33], statements simulated with different speech-encoding strategies differentiated the P200 in the happy expression and an early (0–400 ms) and late (600–1200 ms) gamma band power increase in vocal expressions of happiness, anger, and neutral. In Agrawal et al. [34], the P200 was differentiated by different simulation strategies in all types of emotions, and was larger in happiness than in other emotion types across speech-encoding strategies. These studies emphasized the importance of vocoded simulation to better understand the prosodic cues which cochlear impairment users may be utilizing to decode emotion in the voice. Further studies will also draw upon the merits of multimodal recording and synchronization of neurophysiological and peripheral physiological responses to decoding vocal expressions, including eye movement, pupil dilation, heart rate tracking, etc., to understand how different systems support the understanding of social and emotional information in speech and vocalizations.

Acknowledgements

Special thanks to Professor Dr. Marc D. Pell who leads the Neuropragmatics and Emotion Lab in the School of Communication Sciences and Disorders, the McLaughlin Scholarship and McGill MedStar by Faculty of Medicine, McGill University that were awarded to the author.

Author details

Xiaoming Jiang

Address all correspondence to: xiaoming.jiang@mail.mcgill.ca

School of Communication Sciences and Disorders, Neuropragmatics and Emotion Lab (Pell Lab), Faculty of Medicine, McGill University, Montréal, Canada

References

[1] Kotz, S. A., & Paulmann, S. (2007). When emotional prosody and semantics dance cheek to cheek: ERP evidence. *Brain Research, 1151*(1), 107–118. http://doi.org/10.1016/j.brainres.2007.03.015

[2] Schirmer, A., & Kotz, S. (2006). Beyond the right hemispehre: Brain mechnisms mediating vocal emotional processing. *Trends in Cognitive Sciences, 10,* 24–30. http://dx.doi.org/10.1016/j.tics.2005.11.009

[3] Paulmann, S., & Kotz, S. A. (2008). An ERP investigation on the temporal dynamics of emotional prosody and emotional semantics in pseudo- and lexical-sentence context. *Brain and Language, 105*(1), 59–69. http://doi.org/10.1016/j.bandl.2007.11.005

[4] Rigoulot. S., Pell, M. D., & Armony, J. L. (2015). Time course of the influence of musical expertise on the processing of vocal and musical sounds. *Neuroscience, 290,* 175–184.

[5] Kotz, S., & Paulmann, S. (2011). Emotion, language and the brain. *Language and Linguistic Compass, 5,* 108–125. doi: 10.1111/j.1749-818X.2010.00267.x

[6] Paulmann, S., Bleichner, M., Kotz, S. (2013). Valence, arousal, and task effects in emotional prosody processing. *Frontiers in Psychology, 4,* 345. doi: 10.3389/fpsyg.2013.00345.

[7] Liu, T., Pinheiro, A. P., Deng, G., Nestor, P. G., McCarley, R. W., & Niznikiewicz, M. A. (2012). Electrophysiological insights into processing nonverbal emotional vocalizations. *NeuroReport, 23*(2), 108–112. http://doi.org/10.1097/WNR.0b013e32834ea757

[8] Schirmer, A., Chen, C., Ching, A., Tan, L., Hong, R. (2013). Vocal emotions influence verbal memory: Neural correlates and interindividual differences. *Cognitive, Affective and Behavioral Neuroscience, 13*, 80–93.

[9] Van Overwalle, F., Van den Eede, S., Baetens, K., Vandekerckhove, M. (2009). Trait inferences in goal-directed behavior: ERP timing and localization under spontaneous and intentional processing. *Social, Cognitive & Affective Neuroscience, 4*, 177–190. doi: 10.1093/scan/nsp003.

[10] Pell, M. D., Paulmann, S., Dara, C., Alasseri, A., & Kotz, S. A. (2009). Factors in the recognition of vocally expressed emotions: A comparison of four languages. *Journal of Phonetics, 37*, 417–435. doi:10.1016/j.wocn.2009.07.005

[11] Pell, M. D., Rothermich, K., Liu, P., Paulmann, S., Sethi, S., & Rigoulot, S. (2015). Preferential decoding of emotion from human non-linguistic vocalizations versus speech prosody. *Biological Psychology, 111*, 14–25. http://doi.org/10.1016/j.biopsycho.2015.08.008

[12] Chen, X., Yang, J., Gan, S., & Yang, Y. (2012). The contribution of sound intensity in vocal emotion perception: Behavioral and electrophysiological evidence. *PLoS ONE, 7*(1), e30278. http://doi.org/10.1371/journal.pone.0030278

[13] Wickens, S., & Perry, C. (2015). What do you mean by that?! An electrophysiological study of emotional and attitudinal prosody. *PLoS ONE, 10*(7), 1–24. http://doi.org/10.1371/journal.pone.0132947

[14] Rigoulot. S., Fish. K., & Pell, M. D. (2014). Neural correlates of inferring speaker sincerity from white lies: An event-related potential source localization study. *Brain Research, 1565*, 48–62. http://dx.doi.org/10.1016/j.brainres.2014.04.022

[15] Jiang, X., & Pell, M. D. (2015). On how the brain decodes vocal cues about speaker confidence. *Cortex, 66*, 9–34. http://dx.doi.org/10.1016/j.cortex.2015.02.002

[16] Jiang, X., & Pell, M. D. (2016). Neural responses towards a speaker's feeling of (un)knowing. *Neuropsychologia*, 81, 79–93. http://dx.doi.org/10.1016/j.neuropsychologia.2015.12.008

[17] Jiang, X., & Pell, M. D. (2016).The feeling of another's knowing: How "mixed messages" in speech are reconciled. *Journal of Experimental Psychology:Human Perception and Performance. 42*(9), 1412–1428. http://dx.doi.org/10.1037/xhp0000240

[18] Liu, T., Pinheiro, A., Zhao, Z., Nestor, P. G., McCarley, R. W., & Niznikiewicz, M. A. (2012). Emotional cues during simultaneous face and voice processing: Electrophysiological insights. *PLoS ONE, 7*(2), e31001. http://doi.org/10.1371/journal.pone.0031001

[19] Diamond, E., & Zhang, Y. (2016). Cortical processing of phonetic and emotional information in speech: A cross-modal priming study. *Neuropsychologia, 82*, 110–122. http://doi.org/10.1016/j.neuropsychologia.2016.01.019

[20] Chen, X., Han, L., Pan, Z., Luo, Y., & Wang, P. (2016). Influence of attention on bimodal integration during emotional change decoding: ERP evidence. *International Journal of Psychophysiology, 106*, 14–20. http://doi.org/10.1016/j.ijpsycho.2016.05.009

[21] Chen, X., Pan, Z., Wang, P., Yang, X., Liu, P., You, X., Yuan, J. (2015). The integration of facial and vocal cues during emotional change perception: EEG markers. *Social Cognitive and Affective Neuroscience, 11*(7), 1152–1161. http://doi.org/10.1093/scan/nsv083

[22] Chen, X., Zhao, L., Jiang, A., & Yang, Y. (2011). Event-related potential correlates of the expectancy violation effect during emotional prosody processing. *Biological Psychology, 86*(3), 158–167. http://doi.org/10.1016/j.biopsycho.2010.11.004

[23] Chronaki, G., Broyd, S., Garner, M., Hadwin, J. A., Thompson, M. J. J., & Sonuga-Barke, E. J. S. (2012). Isolating N400 as neural marker of vocal anger processing in 6–11-year old children. *Developmental Cognitive Neuroscience, 2*(2), 268–276. http://doi.org/10.1016/j.dcn.2011.11.007

[24] Grossmann, T. (2015). The development of social brain functions in infancy. *Psychological Bulletin, 141*(6), 1266–1287. http://doi.org/10.1037/bul0000002

[25] Liu, P., Rigoulot, S., & Pell, M. D. (2015). Culture modulates the brain response to human expressions of emotion: Electrophysiological evidence. *Neuropsychologia, 67*, 1–13. http://doi.org/10.1016/j.neuropsychologia.2014.11.034

[26] Liu, P., Rigoulot, S., & Pell, M. D. (2015). Cultural differences in on-line sensitivity to emotional voices: Comparing East and West. *Frontiers in Human Neuroscience, 9*(May), 311. http://doi.org/10.3389/fnhum.2015.00311

[27] Schirmer, A., Kotz, S. (2003). ERP evidence for a sex-specific stroop effect in emotional speech. *Journal of Cognitive Neuroscience, 15*, 1135–1148. doi:10.1162/089892903322598102

[28] Schirmer, A., Kotz, S., Friederici, A. D. (2005). On the role of attention for the processing of emotions in speech. *Cognitive Brain Research, 24*, 442–452. doi:10.1016/j.cogbrainres.2005.02.022

[29] Davis, M. (1983). Measuring individual differences in empathy: Evidence for a multidimensional approach. *Journal of Personality and Social Psychology, 44*, 113–126. http://dx.doi.org/10.1037/0022-3514.44.1.113

[30] Campanella, S., Bruyer, R., Froidbise, S., Rossignol, M., Joassin, F., Kornreich, C., &Verbanck, P. (2010). Is two better than one? A cross-modal oddball paradigm reveals greater sensitivity of the P300 to emotional face-voice associations. *Clinical Neurophysiology, 121*(11), 1855–1862. http://doi.org/10.1016/j.clinph.2010.04.004

[31] Chen, C., Liu, C.-C., Weng, P.-Y., & Cheng, Y. (2016). Mismatch negativity to threatening voices associated with positive symptoms in schizophrenia. *Frontiers in Human Neuroscience , 10*(July), 1–11. http://doi.org/10.3389/fnhum.2016.00362

[32] Lu, X., Ho, H. T., Liu, F., Wu, D., & Thompson, W. F. (2015). Intonation processing deficits of emotional words among Mandarin Chinese speakers with congenital amusia: An ERP study. *Frontiers in Psychology, 6*(March), 1–12. http://doi.org/10.3389/fpsyg.2015.00385

[33] Agrawal, D., Thorne, J., Viola, F., Timm, L., Debener, S., Büchner, A., Dengler, R., Wittfoth, M. (2013). Electrophysiological responses to emotional prosody perception in cochlear implant users. *NeuroImage: Clinical. 2*, 229–238.

[34] Agrawal, D., Timm, L., Viola, F., Debener, S., Büchner, A., Dengler, R., Wittfoth, M. (2012). ERP evidence for the recognition of emotional prosody through simulated cochlear implant strategies. *BMC Neuroscience, 13*, 113.

Chapter 5

Multimodal Affect Recognition: Current Approaches and Challenges

Hussein Al Osman and Tiago H. Falk

Additional information is available at the end of the chapter

http://dx.doi.org/10.5772/65683

Abstract

Many factors render multimodal affect recognition approaches appealing. First, humans employ a multimodal approach in emotion recognition. It is only fitting that machines, which attempt to reproduce elements of the human emotional intelligence, employ the same approach. Second, the combination of multiple-affective signals not only provides a richer collection of data but also helps alleviate the effects of uncertainty in the raw signals. Lastly, they potentially afford us the flexibility to classify emotions even when one or more source signals are not possible to retrieve. However, the multimodal approach presents challenges pertaining to the fusion of individual signals, dimensionality of the feature space, and incompatibility of collected signals in terms of time resolution and format. In this chapter, we explore the aforementioned challenges while presenting the latest scholarship on the topic. Hence, we first discuss the various modalities used in affect classification. Second, we explore the fusion of modalities. Third, we present publicly accessible multimodal datasets designed to expedite work on the topic by eliminating the laborious task of dataset collection. Fourth, we analyze representative works on the topic. Finally, we summarize the current challenges in the field and provide ideas for future research directions.

Keywords: affect recognition, multimodal, machine learning, sensor fusion

1. Introduction

Humans employ rich emotional communication channels during social interaction by modulating their speech utterances, facial expressions, and body gestures. They also rely on emotional cues to resolve the semantics of received messages. Interestingly, humans also communicate emotional information when interacting with machines. They express affects and respond emotionally during human-machine interaction. However, machines, from the simplest to the most intelligent ones devised by humans, have conventionally been completely oblivious to emotional information. This reality is changing with the advent of affective computing.

Affective computing advocates the idea of emotionally intelligent machines. Hence, these machines can recognize and simulate emotions. In fact, over the last decade, we have witnessed a steadily increasing interest in the development of automated methods for human-affect estimation. The applications of such technologies are varied and span several domains. Rosalind Picard, in her 1997 book Affective Computing, describes various applications, such as a computer tutor that personalizes learning based on the user's affective response, affective agent that assists autistic individuals navigate difficult social situations, and a classroom barometer that informs the teacher of the level of engagement of the students [1]. Numerous other applications have been proposed over the years. For instance, many researchers suggest the creation of emotionally intelligent computers to improve the quality of the human-computer interaction (HCI) [2–4]. Other affective computing applications abound in the literature. For example, Gilleade et al. [5] propose the use of affective methods in video gaming. Al Osman et al. [6] present a mobile application for stress management. However, regardless of the application, all researchers in the field are faced with the following questions: How can a machine classify human emotions? What should the machine do in response to the recognized emotions? In this chapter, we are solely concerned with the first question.

Various strategies of affect classification have been successfully employed under restricted circumstances. The primary modalities that have been thoroughly explored pertain to facial-expression estimation, speech-prosody (tone) analysis, physiological signal interpretation, and body-gesture examination. In this chapter, we explore affect-recognition techniques that integrate multiple modalities of affect expression. These techniques are known in the literature as multimodal methods.

Although, today, most of the affective computing applications are unimodal, the multimodal approach has been advocated by numerous researchers [4, 7–14]. There are many reasons that render the multimodal approach appealing. First, humans employ a multimodal approach in emotion recognition. It is only fitting that machines, which attempt to reproduce elements of human emotional intelligence, employ the same approach. Second, the combination of multiple-affective signals not only provides a richer collection of data but also helps alleviate the effects of uncertainty in the raw signals. After all, these signals are collected by imperfect sensors with numerous possible sources of error between the signal producer and processor. Lastly, it potentially gives us the flexibility to classify emotions even when one or more source signals are not possible to retrieve. This can happen in situations where the face or body is partially or fully occluded, which disqualifies the visual modality, or when the user is not speaking which eliminates the vocal modality from consideration. However, the multimodal approach presents challenges pertaining to the fusion of individual signals, dimensionality of the feature space, and incompatibility of collected signals in terms of time resolution and format.

Before we proceed, we clarify a potential source of confusion. The terms affect and emotion can have different meanings in various fields. For instance, according to Shouse, a researcher in communication, an emotion refers to the display of a feeling, whether it is genuine or feigned [15]. However, an "affect is a non-conscious experience of intensity" [15]. Some psychologists consider affect as the experience of emotion [16]. In this chapter, we consider the terms emotion and affect to be synonymous since a sizable amount of works in affective computing use them interchangeably.

The remainder of this chapter is organized as follows: Section 2 summarizes the modalities of affect recognition, Section 3 describes pertinent modality-fusion techniques, Section 4 presents publicly available multimodal emotional databases, Section 5 surveys representative multimodal affect-recognition methods, and Section 6 discusses the challenges in the field and future research directions.

2. Modalities of affect recognition

In this section, we explore the various modalities of emotional channels that can be used for the automated resolution of human affect. The fundamental question that this section addresses is the following: What measurable information the machine needs to retrieve and interpret to estimate human affect?

When it comes to judging expressive behaviors, humans rely in general on verbal and nonverbal channels [17]. The verbal channels correspond to speech, while nonverbal channels include the eye gaze and blink, facial and body expression, and speech prosody. Note that speech corresponds to the semantics of the communicated message while speech prosody is concerned with the tonal content of voice regardless of the meaning of spoken phrases. Facial expression and speech prosody are believed to be the most relied upon by humans for emotions' interpretation [18]. Hence, these channels are likely rich in informational cues about the affective state. Social psychologists have interestingly remarked that expressive behaviors can be consciously regulated to convey a calculated self-presentation. However, nonverbal channels tend to be less vulnerable to deliberate manipulation. Moreover, when verbal behavior conflicts with nonverbal comportment, nonverbal expressions may be more reflective of the true affective status [17]. In fact, researchers have found speech prosody to be the least consciously controllable modality [19]. The latter finding can inform the development of affective applications for lie detection. In the following subsections, we detail the commonly used modalities of affect recognition.

2.1. Visual modalities

The visual modality is rich in relevant informational content and includes the facial expression, eye gaze, pupil diameter, and blinking behavior, and body expression. We explore these affective sources in this section.

2.1.1. *Facial expression*

The most studied nonverbal affect-recognition method is facial-expression analysis [20]. Perhaps, that is because facial expressions are the most intuitive indicators of affect. Even as children, we draw simplistic faces that convey various emotions by manipulating the forehead creases, eyebrows, and mouth. We also find it instinctive to use emoticons in digital textual communications that convey emotions through simple facial-expression depictions.

2.1.1.1. *Facial muscle movement coding*

Facial expressions result from the contraction of facial muscles resulting in the temporary deformation of the neutral expression. These deformations are typically brief and last mostly between 250 ms and 5 s [21]. Darwin [22] is one of the early researchers to explore the evolutionary foundation of facial-expressions display. He argues that facial expressions are universal across humans. He contends that they are habitual movements associated with certain states of the mind. These habits have been favored through natural selection and inherited across generations. Ekman and Fiesen [23] built on the idea of facial-expression universality to conceive the facial action coding system (FACS) that describes all possible perceivable facial muscle movements in terms of predefined action units (AUs). All AUs are numerically coded and facial expressions correspond to one or more AUs. Although FACS is primarily employed to detect emotions, it can be used to describe facial muscle activation regardless of the underlying cause. Inspired by FACS, other facial expression coding systems have been proposed, such as the emotional facial action coding system (EMFACS) [24], the maximally descriptive facial movement coding system (MAX) [25], and the system for identifying affect expressions by holistic judgment AFFEX [26]. The latter systems are solely directed at emotion recognition.

The Moving Pictures Experts Group (MPEG) defined the facial animation parameters (FAPs) in the MPEG-4 standard to enable the animation of face models. MPEG-4 describes facial feature points (FPs) that are controlled by FAPs. The value of the FAP corresponds to the magnitude of deformation of the facial model in comparison to the neutral state. Though the standard was not originally intended for automated emotion detection, it has been employed for that goal in various works [27, 28]. These coding systems inspired researchers to develop automated image or video-processing methods that track the movement of facial features to resolve the affective state [29].

2.1.1.2. *Facial-expression detection*

Facial-expression detection algorithms involve the following three steps: (1) face detection (or face tracking across video frames), (2) feature extraction, and (3) affect classification. We will not discuss face detection or tracking in this chapter, the reader can refer to the plethora of existing literature on the topic (e.g., [30–32]).

Feature extraction is an essential aspect of expression recognition. Jiang et al. [33] divide the feature extraction methods into two types: geometric-based and appearance-based methods. Geometric features typically correspond to the distances between key facial points or the velocity vectors of these points as the facial expression develops. However, appearance features reflect the changes in image texture resulting from the deformation of the neutral expression (e.g., facial bulges and creases) [33]. We detail few feature extraction schemes employed across many works. Each technique listed represents a set of methods that apply the same basic idea in feature extraction:

- Motion estimators: They are geometric-based feature extraction methods. They estimate the motion between two images. The most commonly used algorithm is optical flow [34]. When the latter is used for facial feature extraction, the camera is usually assumed to be stationary and the nonrigid motion resulting from facial deformation is tracked across video frames. The output is a series of vectors that represent motion. This technique has been used in numerous works, either alone [35–37], or in combination with other feature extraction techniques [38].
- Point trackers: They are geometric-based feature extraction methods. They track feature points across an image sequence. A typical algorithm, known as the Kanade-Lucas-Tomasi (KLT) tracker [39, 40], computes the spatial translation or affine transformation of features between consecutive video frames. Spatiotemporal vectors can be obtained from the movement of tracked features.
- Gabor wavelets: They are appearance-based feature extraction methods. They typically use a set of Gabor filters at different scales and orientation for feature extraction. Gabor filters are a type of band-pass filters that act in a similar manner to the human cortical cells by mostly resolving edges of objects present in an image. This technique usually involves training a machine-learning model using Gabor features extracted from a database of facial expression and running the model to classify emotions from images.

For classification, numerous techniques have been proposed such as support vector machine (SVM), neural network (NN), and hidden Markov models (HMMs) [29, 35, 41–45].

In addition to facial-expression analysis, eye-based features such as pupil diameter, gaze distance, and gaze coordinates, and blinking behavior have been used in multimodal systems [10, 12]. In fact, Panning et al. [10] found that in their multimodal system, the speech paralinguistic features and eye-blinking frequency were the most contributing modalities to the classification process.

2.1.2. Body expression

The importance of body expressions for affect recognition has been debated in the literature, with conflicting opinions. McNeill [46] maintains that two-handed gestures are closely associated with the spoken verbs. Hence, they arguably do not present new affective information; they simply accompany the speech modality. Consequently, some researchers argue that gestures may play a secondary role in the human recognition of emotions [4, 13]. This suggests that they might be less reliable than other modalities in delivering affective cues that can be automatically analyzed. However, increasingly, there is more evidence toward the viability of this method in affect recognition, at least for a subset of affective expressions [20, 47–51].

In fact, Lhommet and Marsella [52] contend that body expressions are harder to control consciously than facial expressions, and therefore might reflect more genuine emotions.

Affect recognition using body expression involves tracking the motion of body features in space. Many works rely on the use of three-dimensional (3D) measurement systems that require markers to be attached to the subject's body [11, 53–56]. However, some markerless solutions involving video cameras [57, 58] and wearable sensors [59] have been proposed. Once the motion is captured, a variety of features are extracted from body movement. In particular, the following features have been reliably used: velocity of the body or body part [11, 53, 55, 60–64], acceleration of the body or body part [11, 55, 60, 61, 64], amount of movement [11, 64], joint positions [62], nature of movement (e.g., contraction, expansion, and upward movement) [11], orientation of body parts (e.g., head and shoulder) [54, 56, 63, 64], and angle or distance between body parts (e.g., distance from hand to shoulder and angle between shoulder-shoulder vectors) [54, 56, 61, 63]. Using these features, a variety of classification models have been suggested, such as decision tree [11], multilayered perceptron (MLP) [53, 59], SVM [55, 61, 63], naïve Bayes [63], and HMM [62].

2.2. Audio modality

Speech carries two interrelated informational channels: linguistic information that express the semantics of the message and implicit paralinguistic information conveyed through prosody. Both of these channels carry affective information. Hence, in this section, we briefly describe the general mechanisms of extracting affect from these channels.

2.2.1. Linguistic speech channel

Humans often explain how they feel during social interaction. Hence, building an understanding of the spoken message provides a straightforward way of assessing affect. This technique of affect recognition falls under the wider topic of sentiment analysis and opinion mining using natural language processing. Typically, an automatic speech recognition algorithm is used to convert speech into a textual message. Then, a sentiment analysis method interprets the polarity or emotional content of the message. However, this approach for affect recognition has its pitfalls. First, it is not universal, and therefore a natural language speech processor has to be developed for each dialect; second, it is vulnerable to masking since humans are not always forthcoming about their emotional status [17].

In this section, we only discuss sentiment analysis. We will not cover automatic speech recognition. The readers can consult the survey of Benzeghiba et al. [65] for a thorough treatment of this topic. Sentiment analysis methods can broadly be divided into two categories: lexicon-based techniques and statistical-learning approaches. Lexicon-based techniques classify affect based on the presence of unambiguous affect words or phrases in the text. Numeric values are tied to these words or phrases. Hence, overall sentiment can be extracted through a scoring system that results from the aggregation of these values. Statistical-learning methods, in turn, generate a bag of words whose elements are used as features in machine-learning algorithms. Hybrid approaches that propose a combination of these techniques have also been studied [66, 67].

2.2.2. *Paralinguistic speech-prosody channel*

Sometimes, it is not about what we say, but how we say it. Therefore, speech-prosody analyzers ignore the meaning of messages and focus on acoustic cues that reflect emotions. Before the extraction of tonal features from speech, preprocessing is often necessary to enhance, denoise, and dereverberate the source signal [68]. Then, using windowing functions, low-level descriptor (LLDs) features are extracted at usually 100 frames per second with segment sizes between 10 and 30 ms. Windowing functions are usually rectangular for time-domain features and smooth for frequency or time-frequency features. Numerous LLDs can be extracted, and we list a few: pitch (fundamental frequency F_0), energy (e.g., maximum, minimum, and root mean square), linear prediction cepstral (LPC) coefficients, perceptual linear prediction coefficients, cepstral coefficients (e.g., mel-frequency cepstral coefficients, MFCCs), formants (e.g., amplitude, position, and width), and spectrum (mel-frequency and FFT bands) [68–72]. Linguistic LLDs can also be retrieved, such as word and phoneme sequences [68, 69]. Recently, speech-modulation spectral features were also shown to contain complementary information to prosodic and cepstral features [73].

For classification, global statistics features are classified using static classifier such as SVM [69, 74–76]. Short-term features are processed though dynamic classifiers, such as HMM [68, 76]. Due to the large number of possible features, researchers have proposed the use of dimension-reduction schemes such as principal component analysis (PCA) [69] or linear discriminant analysis (LDA) [68]. More recently, with the burgeoning of deep-learning principles, deep neural networks have also been explored for speech emotion recognition, with very promising results (e.g., [77–79]).

2.3. Physiological modality

Physiological signals can be used for affect recognition through the detection of biological patterns that are reflective of emotional expressions. These signals are collected through typically noninvasive sensors that are affixed to the body of the subject. However, brain imaging [80] and remote physiological monitoring schemes [81, 82] have been proposed.

There are a multitude of physiological signals that can be analyzed for affect detection. Typical physiological signals used for the assessment of affect are electrocardiography (ECG), electromyography (EMG), electroencephalograph (EEG), skin conductance (also known as galvanic skin response, and electrodermal activity), respiration rate, and skin temperature. ECG records the electrical activity of the heart. Conventionally, 12 electrodes are connected to various parts of the body to conduct this measurement. However, in affective computing, most systems use the Lead I configuration that requires only two electrodes [6]. From the ECG signal, the heart rate (HR) and heart rate variability (HRV) can be extracted. HRV is used in numerous studies that assess mental stress [6, 83–85]. EMG measures muscle activity and is known to reflect negatively valenced emotions [86]. EEG is the electrical activity of the brain measured through electrodes connected to the scalp and possibly forehead. There is little agreement on the number of electrodes to use or features to extract from EEG. EEG features are often used to classify emotional dimensions of arousal [87–90], valence [88–90], and dominance [90, 91]. Skin conductance measures the resistance of the skin by passing a negligible current through the body. The resulting signal is reflective of arousal [86] as it corresponds to the activity of the sweat glands. The latter are controlled by the autonomous nervous system (ANS) that regulates the flight or fight response. Finally, respiration rate tends to reflect arousal [92], while skin temperature carries valence cues [93].

3. Multimodal fusion techniques

With multimodal affect-recognition approaches, information extracted from each modality must be reconciled to obtain a single-affect classification result. This is known as multimodal fusion. The literature on this topic is rich and generally describes three types of fusion mechanisms: feature-level fusion, decision-level fusion, and hybrid approaches. In this section, we present the general principles behind these techniques and describe key ideas related to each type.

3.1. Feature-level fusion

A common method to perform modality fusion is to create a single set from all collected features. A single classifier is then trained on the feature set. This method is advocated by Pantic et al. [4, 13] as it mimics the human mechanism of tightly integrating information collected through various sensory channels. However, feature-level fusion is plagued by several challenges. First, the larger multimodal feature set contains more information than the unimodal one. This can present difficulties if the training dataset is limited. Hughes [94] has proven that the increase in the feature set may decrease classification accuracy if the training set is not large enough. Second, features from various modalities are collected at different time scales [13]. For example, frequency domain HRV features typically summarize seconds or minutes' worth of data [6], while speech features can be in the order of milliseconds [13]. Third, a large feature set undoubtedly increases the computational load of the classification algorithm [95]. Finally, one of the advantages of multimodal affect recognition is the ability to produce an emotion classification result in the presence of missing or corrupted data. However, feature-level fusion is more vulnerable to the latter issues than decision-level fusion techniques [96].

3.2. Decision-level fusion

Typically, a classifier makes errors in some area of the feature space [97]. Hence, combining the results of multiple classifiers can alleviate this shortcoming. This is especially true when each classifier is operating on a different modality that corresponds to a separate feature space.

Using decision-level fusion, modalities can be independently classified using separate models and the results are joined using a multitude of possible methods. Therefore, this approach is said to employ an ensemble of classifiers. Ensemble members can belong to the same family or different families of statistical classifiers. In fact, static and dynamic classifiers can both be employed in such a multimodal system.

3.2.1. Combination strategies based on voting

The simplest and one of the oldest methods to achieve decision-level fusion is to use a voting mechanism [98]. Hence, the classification reached by the majority of the ensemble members is adopted as the outcome. However, a tie in the votes can be reached if the number of classifiers is odd. This disqualifies bimodal affect-recognition systems. Furthermore, even for an odd number of classifiers, a definite decision cannot be guaranteed if more than two classes are being considered [95] (e.g., the six prototypical emotions). The classification of a single affect is a typical binary problem that can be solved using this approach. A system that monitors a single affect such as stress or frustration can use this approach as long as an odd number of modalities are supported.

3.2.2. Combination strategies based on prior knowledge

In many cases, it is crucial to assess the performance of each classifier to inform decision making during the combination process. For instance, using the training dataset, we can calculate the confusion matrix for each classifier. Given an ensemble of C classifiers, the confusion matrix of classifier c_i, where $i = 1..C$, is described by

$$Pc_i = \begin{bmatrix} n^i_{11} & \cdots & n^i_{1M} \\ \vdots & \ddots & \vdots \\ n^i_{M1} & \cdots & n^i_{MM} \end{bmatrix} \tag{1}$$

where njki corresponds to the number of times c_i classified an observed sample x as belonging to class r_j while in reality it belongs to class r_k, and M is the total number of classes. The diagonal of the confusion matrix where $j = k$ represents the times where the classifier was correct.

To overcome the limitations of the voting approach, a weighted majority voting scheme can be used. In this approach, classifiers are not treated as equal peers and their votes are weighted to reduce the probability of a tie. The weights can be calculated based on the performance of the classifier in terms of recognition and error rates retrieved from the confusion matrix during training or using a test dataset after training [95, 98, 99]. Lam and Suen [99] propose an optimization process that uses a genetic algorithm to compute the voting weights. They observe that there is often a trade-off between recognition, rejection, and error rates. Therefore, they attempt to maximize objective function (1):

$$F = \text{recognition} - \beta \times \text{error} \tag{2}$$

where β is a constant that can take on different values depending on the accuracy and reliability desired [99]. Hence, in the genetic algorithm, F is used as the fitness value.

Beyond the use of voting schemes, Huang and Suen [100] use a lookup table during training to keep track of the combinations of classifier outputs along with the correct class and number of occurrence of this combination. The number of occurrence reflects the confidence level that the corresponding combination produces the recorded correct class. When the latter combination is observed, the outcome with the highest confidence level, as recorded in the lookup table, is chosen. Gupta et al., in turn, proposed a quality-aware decision fusion scheme, where classifiers were developed for several physiological modalities (i.e., EEG, ECG, GSR, and facial features) and their individual decisions were weighted by the measured quality of each raw signal [101]. Experimental results showed that system failure rates due to noisy segments were drastically reduced, and improved affect-recognition performance could be achieved [101].

Kim and Lingenfelser [102] introduce an ensemble combination strategy that accounts for the capability of some ensemble members to classify certain classes better than others. Therefore, they rank the classes according to the accuracy of their classification across all ensemble members using the confusion matrices produced from the training data. To reach an ensemble decision for an observed sample, the classifier corresponding to the highest-ranked class performs the classification. We refer to that class as the test class. If the classification result matches the test class, then that result is taken to be the ensemble decision. If not, then the next class in the ranked list becomes the test class and the procedure is repeated. If we do not obtain a match for any of the classes, then the classifier with the best overall performance on the training data is tasked with the classification on behalf of the ensemble.

Lastly, Gupta, Laghari, and Falk have made use of a variant of the SVM called relevance vector machines (RVMs) for affect recognition. RVMs have the same functional form of SVMs but are embedded into a Bayesian framework [103]. Therefore, for classification, RVMs compute the probabilities of class membership rather than the point estimates. These class membership probabilities can be seen as a measure of classifier "confidence" and were used as weights for decision-level fusion [90]. While the work in [90] focuses only on a single modality, EEG, it fused the decisions of classifiers trained on different classes of EEG features (power spectral, asymmetry, and graph theoretic), and thus the observed advantages could also be seen for multimodal setups.

3.2.3. Combination strategies for continuous output classifiers

For the ensemble decision of continuous output problems, the probabilities for each class over all classifiers can be used for fusion. Lingenfelser et al. [95] refer to this probability as support and we adopt this terminology. Using these probabilities, several decision-level combination rules are conceived. We detail only a subset of these rules. The maximum rule stipulates that the ensemble decision for an observed feature vector corresponds to the class with the largest support. The sum rule sums the total support for each class chosen by any of the classifiers. Then, the class with the largest support is chosen as the ensemble decision. Similarly, the mean rule calculates the mean support for each chosen class as opposed to the sum. Instead of calculating the mean, a weighted average of total support for each chosen class can also be calculated. Finally, the product rule is similar to the sum rule, except for the use of the multiplication operation instead of the addition for the calculation of the total support.

3.3. Hybrid fusion

When a fusion technique combines feature and decision-level fusion, it is referred to as a hybrid-fusion scheme. For instance, we can achieve fusion in two stages. In the first stage, a classifier can perform feature-level fusion. For example, a single classifier can handle features from audio and video signals. In the second stage, decision-level fusion can be used to combine the results of that classifier with another one operating on physiological (e.g., HRV) features.

Ref. [104] proposes a simple hybrid-fusion approach where the result from the feature-level fusion is fed as an additional input to the decision-level fusion stage. Lingenfelser et al. [95]

propose two variants of one method called the one versus rest. This approach creates an ensemble composed of classifiers trained on each feature set (i.e., features from a modality). However, these classifiers model a two-class problem. That is, each one of them is specialized in classifying a single class. One last multiclass classifier is added to the ensemble and is trained on the merged feature set (i.e., features from all modalities). For the first variant, during classification, for an observed sample, the support for a class obtained from its two-class classifiers is multiplied with the support of the multiclass classifier to obtain an accumulated support. The class with the highest accumulated support is chosen as the ensemble decision. The second variant is similar, except that it chooses the best two-class classifier for each class and uses it to calculate accumulated support.

3.4. Dimensionality problem

Affective information tends to be highly dimensional. It is not unusual for a feature set to contain thousands of variables. Valstar and Pantic [105] model the facial action temporal dynamics by extracting 2520 features from each facial video frame. The problem can be further exasperated when multiple modalities are considered. Feature-level fusion techniques are especially vulnerable to this problem. For instance, Kim and Lingenfelser [102] extract 1280 speech and 26 physiological features to classify affect. Two strategies are generally adopted to reduce the feature space dimension. First, feature-selection techniques that choose a subset of the feature set for model construction are widely used [7, 12, 28, 104]. Second, dimension-reduction methods such as principal component analysis and linear discriminant analysis are commonly employed [7, 10, 106].

4. Multimodal datasets

One of the challenges in developing multimodal affect-recognition methods is the need to collect multisensory data from a large number of subjects. Also, it is difficult to compare the obtained results with other studies given that the experimental setup varies. Therefore, it is essential to use databases to streamline research efforts on the topic and produce repeatable and easy-to-compare results. Very few multimodal affect databases are publicly available. We divide these databases into three types: posed, induced, and natural-emotional databases. For the posed databases, the subjects are asked to act out a specific emotion while the result is captured. Typically, facial and body expression and speech information are captured in posed databases. However, posed databases have their limitations, as they cannot incorporate biosignals; it cannot be guaranteed that posed emotions trigger the same physiological response as spontaneous ones [107]. For the induced databases, the subjects are exposed to a stimulus (e.g., watching a video) in a controlled setting, such as laboratory. The stimulus is designed to evoke certain emotions. In some cases, following the stimulus, the subjects are explicitly asked to act out an emotional expression. The eNTERFACE'05 [108] is an example of such database. These databases combine aspects of induced and posed emotions. For the natural databases, the subjects are exposed to a real-life stimulus such as interaction with human or machine. Data collection mostly occurs in a noncontrolled environment. The AFEW database

[109] presents annotated video clips from movies. Therefore, although the emotional expressions are acted out by professional actors, they take place in real-world environments (or at least simulated ones). Since these expressions are likely to be as subtle as naturally occurring ones, as actors strive to mimic realistic behavior, we categorize this database as a natural one. We concede that it does not perfectly fit in any of the three presented types.

For the induced and natural databases, the measured sensory information is labeled with the emotional information. The label is usually obtained through subject self-assessment, observer/listener judgment, or FACS coding (manually coded facial expressions). Self-assessment is performed using tools such as self-assessment Manikin (SAM) [110] or feeltrace [111]. **Table 1** shows a list of publicly accessible multimodal emotional databases. Most of the databases address the visual and audio modalities, while few recent ones introduce physiological channels.

Reference	DB type	# Subjects	Modalities	Affects	Labeling
GEMEP (2012) [112]	Posed	10	Visual and audio	Amusement, pride, joy, relief, interest, pleasure, hot anger, panic fear, despair, irritation, anxiety, sadness, admiration, tenderness, disgust, contempt, and surprise	N/A
SAL (2008) [113]	Induced	24	Visual and audio	Dimensional and categorical labeling	Feeltrace
Belfast (2000) [114]	Natural	24	Visual and audio	Dimensional and categorical labeling	Feeltrace
MIT (2005) [83]	Natural	17	Physiological (ECG, EMG, skin conductance, and respiration)	Low, medium, and high stress	Observers' judgment
HUMAINE (2007) [115]	Induced and natural	Multiple databases	Visual, audio, and physiological (ECG, skin conductance and temperature, and respiration)	Varies across databases	Observers' judgment + self-assessment
VAM (2008) [116]	Natural	19	Visual and audio	Dimensional labeling	SAM
SEMAINE (2010) [117]	Induced	20	Visual and audio	Dimensional labeling and six basic emotions	Observers' judgment
DEAP (2012) [118]	Induced	32	Visual for (22 subjects) and physiological (EEG, ECG, EMG, and skin conductance)	Dimensional labeling	SAM
MAHNOB-HCI (2012) [12]	Induced	27	Visual (face + eye gaze), audio, and physiological (EEG, ECG, skin conductance and temperature, and respiration)	Dimensional and categorical labeling	Self-assessment (SAM for arousal and valence)

Reference	DB type	# Subjects	Modalities	Affects	Labeling
eNTERFACE'05 (2006) [108]	Posed + induced	42	Visual and audio	Six basic emotions	Observers' verification
RECOLA (2013) [119]	Natural	46	Visual, audio, and physiological (ECG and skin conductance)	Dimensional labeling	Observers' judgment
PhySyQX (2015) [120]	Natural	21	Audio and physiological (EEG and near-infrared spectroscopy, NIRS)	Dimensional labeling	SAM (valence, arousal, dominance) plus nine other quality metrics (e.g., naturalness, acceptance)
AFEW (2012) [109]	Natural	N/A(1426 video clips)	Visual and audio	Six basic emotions + neutral	Expressive keywords from movie subtitles + observers' verification

Table 1. Summary of the characteristics of publicly accessible multimodal emotional databases.

5. Multimodal affect detection

Humans display emotions through a variety of behaviors that are difficult for a machine to fully appreciate. They modulate their facial muscles, eye gaze, body gestures, gait, and speech tone among other channels of expression to convey emotions. Therefore, the understanding of these emotional cues requires a multisensory system that is able to track several or all of these channels.

Many multimodal affect-recognition schemes have been proposed. They generally differ in terms of the modalities, classification method, and fusion mechanism used, and emotions recognized. In **Table 2**, we survey several representative multimodal affect-recognition studies. Facial-expression analysis features prominently in these studies, followed by speech prosody. However, there seems to be little agreement on the nature and number of the features to be extracted for each modality.

All of the reviewed works consider a subset of possible features that can be extracted from the dataset. Therefore, effective feature selection is required to simplify the classification models, and reduce training time and overfitting. Hence, diverse automated techniques are employed for that purpose, such as the wrapper method [28], analysis of variance (ANOVA)-based approach [12], sequential backward selection [7], minimum redundancy maximum relevance [121], and correlation-based feature selection [104]. Some works rely on expert knowledge [27, 106] as an effective feature-selection scheme. Furthermore, several works elect to reduce the dimensionality of the feature space using PCA [7, 10, 106].

Reference	Modalities	Classifier**	Features	Affects	DB type	Overall recognition rate*
Castellano et al. [28]	Visual (face, body) and audio	BN	**Face:** statistical values from FAPs and their derivatives **Body:** quantity of motion and contraction index of the body, velocity, acceleration, and fluidity of the hand's barycenter **Speech:** intensity, pitch, MFCC, Bark spectral bands, voiced segment characteristics, and pause length (377 features in total)	Anger, despair, interest, pleasure, sadness, irritation, joy and pride	Posed	FLF: 78.3% DLF: 74.6%
Panning et al. [10]	Visual (face and body) and audio	PCA+MLP	**Face:** eye blink per minute, mouth deformations, eyebrow actions **Body:** touch hand to face (binary) **Speech:** 36 features (12 MFCCs, their deltas and accelerations, and the zero-mean coefficient)	Frustration	Natural	FLF: 40–90%
Busso et al. [7]	Visual (face) and audio	SVM	**Face:** Four-dimensional feature vectors **Speech:** mean, standard deviation, range, maximum, minimum, and median of pitch and intensity	Anger, sadness, happiness, neutral	Posed	FLF: 89.1% DLF: 89.0%
Kapoor et al. [123]	Visual (face, posture) and physiological	GP	**Face:** nod and shakes, eye blinks, mouth activities, shape of eyes and eyebrows **Posture:** pressure matrices (on chair while seated) **Physiological:** skin conductance **Behavioral:** pressure on mouse	Frustration	Natural	FLF: 79%
Soleymani et al. [12]	Physiological + eye gaze	SVM (RBF Kernel)	**Physiological:** 20 GSR, 63 ECG, 14 respiration, 4 skin temperature, and 216 EEG features **Eye gaze:** pupil diameter, gaze distance, gaze coordinates	Arousal and valence	Induced	DLF: 72%

Reference	Modalities	Classifier**	Features	Affects	DB type	Overall recognition rate*
Kapoor and Picard [9]	Visual (face, and posture) and context	MGP	**Face:** Five features from upper face and two features from lower face **Posture:** current posture and level of activity **Context:** level of difficulty, state of the game	Student interest level	Natural	FLF: 86%
Paleari et al. [14]	Visual (face) and audio	NN	**Face:** 24 features corresponding to 12 pairs of feature points + 14 distance features **Speech:** 26 features, *F0*, formants (*F1–F3*), energy, harmonicity, LPC1 to LPC9, MFCC1 to MFCC10)	Six basic emotions	Induced + posed	DLF: 75%
Kim et al. [104]	Audio and physiological	LDF	**Physiological:** EMG at the nape of the neck, ECG, skin conductance, and respiration (26 features in total) **Speech:** pitch, utterance, energy, and 12 MFCC features	Positive/high, positive/low, negative/high, and negative/low	Induced	DLF: 57% FLF: 66% HF: 60%
Lin et al. [27]	Visual (face) and audio	C– HMM, SC-HMM, and EWSC-HMM	**Face:** FAPs calculated from 68 feature points on eyebrows, eyes, nose, mouth, and facial contour **Speech:** pitch, energy, and formants (*F1–F5*)	Joy, anger, sadness, and neutral Valence and arousal quadrants	Posed Induced	FLF: 75% DLF: 80% HF: 83–91% FLF: 64% DLF:69% HF: 66–78%
Ringeval et al. [106]	Visual (face), audio, and physiological	SVR + NN	**Face:** 84 appearance based features (after PCA based reduction) obtained from local Gabor binary patterns from three orthogonal planes + 196 geometric features based on 49 tracked facial landmarks **Speech:** One energy, 25 spectral (e.g., MFCC, spectral flux), and 16 voicing (e.g., F0, formants, and jitter) features **Physiological:** ECG (HR + HRV) and skin conductance	Valence and arousal	Natural	DLF: average correlation with self-assessment of 42%
Gupta et al. [101]	Visual (face/ head-pose) and physiological	SVM, NB	**Face/Head-pose:** lips thickness, spatial ratios (e.g., upper to lower lip thickness, eye brows to lips width) **Physiological:** ECG (power spectral features over ECG and HRV), skin conductance (power spectral, zero-crossing rate, rise time, fall time), EEG (band powers for δ-, θ-, α-, β-, and γ-bands)	Valence, arousal, and liking of multimedia content	Natural	DLF: *F1*-score of 59% (SVM) and 57% (NB)

Reference	Modalities	Classifier**	Features	Affects	DB type	Overall recognition rate*
Kaya and Salah [121]	Visual (face) and audio	ELM	**Face:** image is divided into 16 regions. 177 dimensional descriptors are extracted from each region using a local binary pattern histogram **Audio:** 1582 features such as *F0*, MFCC (0–14), and line spectral frequencies (0–7)	Six basic emotions + neutral	Natural	DLF: 44.23%

*FLF: Feature-Level Fusion, DLF: Decision-Level Fusion, HF: Hybrid Fusion.
**HMM: Hidden Markov Mode, C-HMM: Coupled HMM, SC-HMM: Semi-Coupled HMM, EWSC-HMM: Error Weighted SC-HMM, SVR: Support Vector Regression, LDF: Linear Discrimination Function, NN: Neural Networks, GP: Gaussian Process, MGP: Mixture of Gaussian Processes, MLP: Multilayer Perceptron, BN: Bayesian Network, NB: Naïve Bayes. ELM: Extreme Learning Machine.

Table 2. Representative multimodal affect-recognition studies.

Three modality-fusion techniques are commonly employed. There seems to be somewhat conflicting results concerning the most effective class of modality-fusion methods. For instance, Kapoor and Picard [9] obtain better results using feature-level fusion. Conversely, Busso et al. [7] fail to realize a discernible difference between the two methods. Beyond the latter two approaches, Lin et al. [27] propose three hybrid approaches that use coupled HMM, semi-coupled HMM, and error-weighted semi-coupled HMM based on a Bayesian classifier-weighing method. Their results show improvements over feature-and decision-level fusion for posed and induced-emotional databases. However, Kim et al. [104] were not able to improve over decision-level fusion with their proposed hybrid approach. The presence of confounding variables such as modalities, emotions, classification technique, feature selection and reduction approaches, and datasets used limits the value of comparing fusion results across studies. Consequently, Lingenfelser et al. [95] conducted a systematic study of several feature-level, decision-level, and hybrid-fusion techniques for multimodal affect detection. They were not able to find clear advantages for one technique over another.

Various affect classification methods are employed. For dynamic classification where the evolving nature of an observed phenomenon is classified, HMM is the prevalent choice of classifier [27]. For static classification, researchers use a variety of classifiers and we were not able to discern any clear advantages of one over another. However, an empirical study of unimodal affect recognition through physiological features found an advantage for SVM over *k*-nearest neighbor, regression tree, and Bayesian network [122]. Yet, a systematic investigation of the effectiveness of classifiers for multimodal affect recognition is needed to address the issue.

The database type seems to have an effect on the overall affect-recognition rate. We notice that studies that use posed databases generally achieve higher levels of accuracy compared to ones that use other types (e.g., [7, 27]). In fact, Lin et al. [27] perform an analysis of recognition rates using the same methods on two database types: posed and induced. They achieve significantly better results with the posed database. Natural databases result in typically lower recognition rates (e.g., [10, 101, 106, 121]) with the exception of studies [9, 123] that classify a single affect.

http://dx.doi.org/10.5772/65683

6. Discussion and conclusion

In this chapter, we have reviewed and presented the various affect-detection modalities, multimodal affect-recognition schemes, modality-fusion methods, and public multimodal-emotional databases. Although the work on multimodal human-affect classification has been ongoing for years, there are still many challenges to overcome. In this section, we detail these challenges and describe future research directions.

6.1. Current challenges

Numerous studies found multimodal methods to perform as good as or better than unimodal ones [9, 14, 27, 28, 104, 106]. However, the improvements of multimodal systems over unimodal ones are modest when affect detection is performed on spontaneous expressions in natural settings [124]. Also, multimodal methods introduce new challenges that have not been fully resolved. We summarize these challenges as follows:

- Multimodal affect-recognition methods require multisensory systems to collect the relevant data. These systems are more complex than unimodal ones in terms of the number and diversity of sensors involved and the computational complexity of the data-interpreting algorithms. This challenge is more evident when data are collected in a natural setting where user movement is not constrained to a controlled environment. Most physiological sensors are wearable and sensitive to movement. Therefore, additional signal filtering and preparation are required. Audio and visual data quality depends heavily on the distance between the subject and sensors and the presence of occluding objects between them.
- Multimodal affect-recognition methods necessitate the fusion of the modal features extracted from the raw signals. It is still unclear which fusion techniques outperform the others [95]. It seems that the performance of the fusion technique depends on the number of modalities, features extracted, types of classifiers, and the dataset used in the analysis [95]. While the first steps toward a quality-aware fusion system have been proposed [101], more research is still needed in order to gauge the true benefit of such an approach.
- It is still not understood what type and number of modalities are needed to achieve the highest level of accuracy in affect classification. Also, it is unclear how each modality contributes to the effectiveness of the system. Very few studies attempt to test the effect of single modalities on the overall performance [10] and a systematic study of the issue is still required.
- It is well established that context affects how humans express emotions [125, 126]. Nonetheless, context is disregarded by most work on affect recognition [127]. Therefore, we still need to address the challenge of incorporating contextual information into the affect classification process. Some attempts have been done in this regard [9, 123, 128–131]. For instance, Kim [128] suggests a two-stage procedure, where in the first stage, the affective dimensions of valence and arousal are classified, and in the second stage, the uncertainties between adjacent emotions in the two dimensional-affective space are resolved using

contextual information. However, more work is needed to validate this method and propose other similar methods that incorporate a rich set of contextual features.

- Although we have had major improvements in terms of the availability of public multimodal affect datasets over the past few years, many of the works in the area still use private datasets [127]. The use of nonpublic datasets makes results across studies challenging to compare and progress in the field difficult to trace.
- Multimodal-affective systems collect potentially private information such as video and physiological data. Special care needs to be afforded to the protection of such sensitive data. To the best of our knowledge, no work has specifically addressed this issue yet in the context of affective computing.
- In addition to the abundant technical challenges, the ethical implications of designing emotionally intelligent machines and how this can affect the human perception of these machines must be queried.

Despite these challenges, the results achieved in the last decade are very encouraging and the community of researchers on the topic is growing [124].

6.2. Future research directions

Several streams of research are still worth pursuing in the domain. For instance, more investigation is required on the usefulness and applicability of fusion techniques to different modalities and feature sets. Existing studies did not find consistent improvement in the accuracy of affect recognition between feature- and decision-level fusion. However, decision-level fusion schemes are advantageous when it comes to dealing with missing data [96]. After all, multisensory signal collection systems are prone to lost or corrupted segments of data. The introduction of effective hybrid-fusion techniques can further improve accuracy of classification. An empirical and exhaustive study of classifiers in multimodal emotion detection systems is still needed to gain a better understanding about their effectiveness. Although we have seen a flurry of new multimodal emotional databases in the last few years, there is still a need to create richer databases with larger amounts of data and support for more modalities. Moreover, new sensors and wearable technologies are emerging continuously, which may open doors for new affect-recognition modalities. For example, functional near-infrared spectroscopy (fNIRS) has been recently explored within this context [132]. fNIRS, much like functional magnetic resonance imagining (fMRI), measures cerebral blood flow and hemoglobin concentrations in the cortex, but at a fraction of the cost, without the interference of MRI acoustic noise, and with the advantage of being portable. Moreover, recent studies have explored the extraction of physiological information (e.g., heart rate and breathing) from face videos [81, 82], and thus may open doors for multimodal systems, which, in essence, would require only one modality (i.e., video). Notwithstanding, the biggest research challenge that remains is the detection of natural emotions. We have seen in this chapter that the accuracy of detection method decreases when natural emotions are classified. This is mainly due to the subtlety of the natural emotions (compared to exaggerated posed ones) and their dependence on the context [126]. Therefore, we expect that a considerable amount of future research will be dedicated for this effort.

Author details

Hussein Al Osman[1] and Tiago H. Falk[2]*

*Address all correspondence to: falk@emt.inrs.ca

1 University of Ottawa, Ottawa, Ontario, Canada

2 Institut National de la Recherche Scientifique, INRS-EMT, University of Quebec, Montreal, Quebec, Canada

References

[1] R. W. Picard, *Affective computing*. Cambridge, MA: MIT Press, 1997.

[2] R. W. Picard, "Affective computing for HCI," in *HCI*, vol. 1, pp. 829–833, 1999.

[3] T. Partala and V. Surakka, "The effects of affective interventions in human–computer interaction," *Interacting with Computers*, vol. 16, pp. 295–309, 2004.

[4] M. Pantic, N. Sebe, J. F. Cohn, and T. Huang, "Affective multimodal human-computer interaction," in *Proceedings of the 13th annual ACM international conference on multimedia*, 2005, pp. 669–676.

[5] K. Gilleade, A. Dix, and J. Allanson, "Affective videogames and modes of affective gaming: assist me, challenge me, emote me," *Proceedings of DiGRA*, 2005.

[6] H. Al Osman, H. Dong, and A. El Saddik, "Ubiquitous biofeedback serious game for stress management," *IEEE Access*, vol. 4, pp. 1274–1286, 2016.

[7] C. Busso, Z. Deng, S. Yildirim, M. Bulut, C. M. Lee, A. Kazemzadeh, *et al.*, "Analysis of emotion recognition using facial expressions, speech and multimodal information," in *Proceedings of the 6th international conference on multimodal interfaces*, 2004, pp. 205–211.

[8] Z. Zeng, Y. Hu, Y. Fu, T. S. Huang, G. I. Roisman, and Z. Wen, "Audio-visual emotion recognition in adult attachment interview," in *Proceedings of the 8th international conference on multimodal interfaces*, 2006, pp. 139–145.

[9] A. Kapoor and R. W. Picard, "Multimodal affect recognition in learning environments," in *Proceedings of the 13th annual ACM international conference on multimedia*, 2005, pp. 677–682.

[10] A. Panning, I. Siegert, A. Al-Hamadi, A. Wendemuth, D. Rösner, J. Frommer, *et al.*, "Multimodal affect recognition in spontaneous hci environment," in *2012 IEEE international conference on signal processing, communication and computing (ICSPCC)*, 2012, pp. 430–435.

[11] A. Camurri, B. Mazzarino, M. Ricchetti, R. Timmers, and G. Volpe, "Multimodal analysis of expressive gesture in music and dance performances," in *International gesture workshop*, 2003, pp. 20–39.

[12] M. Soleymani, J. Lichtenauer, T. Pun, and M. Pantic, "A multimodal database for affect recognition and implicit tagging," *IEEE Transactions on Affective Computing,* vol. 3, pp. 42–55, 2012.

[13] M. Pantic and L. J. Rothkrantz, "Toward an affect-sensitive multimodal human-computer interaction," *Proceedings of the IEEE,* vol. 91, pp. 1370–1390, 2003.

[14] M. Paleari, B. Huet, and R. Chellali, "Towards multimodal emotion recognition: a new approach," in *Proceedings of the ACM international conference on image and video retrieval,* 2010, pp. 174–181.

[15] E. Shouse, "Feeling emotion affect", *Media Culture Journal,* vol. 8, no. 6, pp. 1, 2005.

[16] M. A. Hogg and D. Abrams, "Social cognition and attitudes," in Martin, G. Neil and Carlson, Neil R. and Buskist, William, eds. *Psychology,* third edition, Pearson Education Limited, 2007, pp. 684–721.

[17] N. Ambady and R. Rosenthal, "Thin slices of expressive behavior as predictors of interpersonal consequences: A meta-analysis," *Psychological Bulletin,* vol. 111, p. 256, 1992.

[18] N. Fragopanagos and J. G. Taylor, "Emotion recognition in human–computer interaction," *Neural Networks,* vol. 18, pp. 389–405, 2005.

[19] R. Rosenthal and B. M. DePaulo, "Sex differences in accommodation in nonverbal communication," In *Skill in nonverbal communication: Individual differences,* Cambridge, MA: Oelgeschlager, Gunn and Hain, 1979, pp. 68–103.

[20] B. de Gelder, "Why bodies? Twelve reasons for including bodily expressions in affective neuroscience," *Philosophical Transactions of the Royal Society B: Biological Sciences,* vol. 364, pp. 3475–3484, 2009.

[21] B. Fasel and J. Luettin, "Automatic facial expression analysis: A survey," *Pattern Recognition,* vol. 36, pp. 259–275, 2003.

[22] C. Darwin, *The expression of the emotions in man and animals,* London, UK: John Murray, 1965.

[23] P. Ekman and W. V. Friesen, "*Facial action coding system,*" Palo Alto: Consulting Psychologists Press, 1978.

[24] W. V. Friesen and P. Ekman, "*EMFACS-7: Emotional facial action coding system,*" Unpublished manuscript, San Francisco: University of California, 1983.

[25] C. E. Izard, "*The maximally discriminative facial movement coding system*", Newark, Canada: Academic Computing Services and University Media Services, University of Delaware, revised edition, 1983.

[26] C. E. Izard, L. M. Dougherty, and E. A. Hembree, "*A system for identifying affect expressions by holistic judgments (AFFEX)*", Instructional Resources Center, University of Delaware, 1983.

[27] J.-C. Lin, C.-H. Wu, and W.-L. Wei, "Error weighted semi-coupled hidden Markov model for audio-visual emotion recognition," *IEEE Transactions on Multimedia,* vol. 14, pp. 142–156, 2012.

http://dx.doi.org/10.5772/65683

[28] G. Castellano, L. Kessous, and G. Caridakis, "Emotion recognition through multiple modalities: face, body gesture, speech," in *Affect and emotion in human-computer interaction*, Berlin Heidelberg, Germany: Springer, 2008, pp. 92–103.

[29] I. Cohen, N. Sebe, A. Garg, L. S. Chen, and T. S. Huang, "Facial expression recognition from video sequences: temporal and static modeling," *Computer Vision and Image Understanding*, vol. 91, pp. 160–187, 2003.

[30] R.-L. Hsu, M. Abdel-Mottaleb, and A. K. Jain, "Face detection in color images," *IEEE Transactions on Pattern Analysis and Machine Intelligence*, vol. 24, pp. 696–706, 2002.

[31] C. Zhang and Z. Zhang, "*A survey of recent advances in face detection*," ed: Tech. rep., Microsoft Research, 2010.

[32] E. Hjelmås and B. K. Low, "Face detection: A survey," *Computer Vision and Image Understanding*, vol. 83, pp. 236–274, 2001.

[33] B. Jiang, M. F. Valstar, and M. Pantic, "Action unit detection using sparse appearance descriptors in space-time video volumes," in *2011 IEEE international conference on automatic face & gesture recognition and workshops (FG 2011)*, 2011, pp. 314–321.

[34] S. S. Beauchemin and J. L. Barron, "The computation of optical flow," *ACM Computing Surveys (CSUR)*, vol. 27, pp. 433–466, 1995.

[35] K. Anderson and P. W. McOwan, "A real-time automated system for the recognition of human facial expressions," *IEEE Transactions on Systems, Man, and Cybernetics, Part B (Cybernetics)*, vol. 36, pp. 96–105, 2006.

[36] Y. Yacoob and L. S. Davis, "Recognizing human facial expressions from long image sequences using optical flow," *IEEE Transactions on Pattern Analysis and Machine Intelligence*, vol. 18, pp. 636–642, 1996.

[37] M. Kenji, "Recognition of facial expression from optical flow," *IEICE Transactions on Information and Systems*, vol. 74, pp. 3474–3483, 1991.

[38] Y.-I. Tian, T. Kanade, and J. F. Cohn, "Recognizing action units for facial expression analysis," *IEEE Transactions on Pattern Analysis and Machine Intelligence*, vol. 23, pp. 97–115, 2001.

[39] B. D. Lucas and T. Kanade, "An iterative image registration technique with an application to stereo vision," in *IJCAI*, 1981, pp. 674–679.

[40] J. Shi and C. Tomasi, "Good features to track," in *1994 IEEE computer society conference on computer vision and pattern recognition, 1994. Proceedings CVPR'94*, 1994, pp. 593–600.

[41] M. Pardàs and A. Bonafonte, "Facial animation parameters extraction and expression recognition using Hidden Markov Models," *Signal Processing: Image Communication*, vol. 17, pp. 675–688, 2002.

[42] P. Michel and R. El Kaliouby, "Real time facial expression recognition in video using support vector machines," in *Proceedings of the 5th international conference on multimodal interfaces*, 2003, pp. 258–264.

[43] I. Kotsia and I. Pitas, "Facial expression recognition in image sequences using geometric deformation features and support vector machines," *IEEE Transactions on Image Processing,* vol. 16, pp. 172–187, 2007.

[44] I. Kotsia, I. Buciu, and I. Pitas, "An analysis of facial expression recognition under partial facial image occlusion," *Image and Vision Computing,* vol. 26, pp. 1052–1067, 2008.

[45] M.S. Bartlett, G. Littlewort, I. Fasel, R. Movellan, "Real time face detection and facial expression recognition: Development and application to human computer interaction", *Proc. CVPR workshop on computer vision and pattern recognition for human-computer interaction*, vol. 5, 2006.

[46] D. McNeill, *Hand and mind: What gestures reveal about thought,* Chicago, IL: University of Chicago Press, 1992.

[47] P. E. Bull, *Posture & gesture,* Oxford, England: Pergamon Press, 1987.

[48] M. Argyle, *Bodily communication* (2nd ed.), London, England: Methuen, 1988.

[49] L. McClenney and R. Neiss, "Posthypnotic suggestion: A method for the study of nonverbal communication," *Journal of Nonverbal Behavior,* vol. 13, pp. 37–45, 1989.

[50] H. K. Meeren, C. C. van Heijnsbergen, and B. de Gelder, "Rapid perceptual integration of facial expression and emotional body language," *Proceedings of the National Academy of Sciences of the United States of America,* vol. 102, pp. 16518–16523, 2005.

[51] J. Van den Stock, R. Righart, and B. De Gelder, "Body expressions influence recognition of emotions in the face and voice," *Emotion,* vol. 7, p. 487, 2007.

[52] Lhommet M., Marsella S.C., "Expressing emotion through posture," In Calvo R., D'Mello S., Gratch J., Kappas A., *The Oxford handbook of affective computing,* Oxford, UK: Oxford University Press, 2014, pp. 273–285.

[53] F. E. Pollick, V. Lestou, J. Ryu, and S.-B. Cho, "Estimating the efficiency of recognizing gender and affect from biological motion," *Vision Research,* vol. 42, pp. 2345–2355, 2002.

[54] A. Kleinsmith and N. Bianchi-Berthouze, "Recognizing affective dimensions from body posture," in *International conference on affective computing and intelligent interaction,* 2007, pp. 48–58.

[55] L. Gong, T. Wang, C. Wang, F. Liu, F. Zhang, and X. Yu, "Recognizing affect from nonstylized body motion using shape of Gaussian descriptors," in *Proceedings of the 2010 ACM symposium on applied computing,* 2010, pp. 1203–1206.

[56] N. Bianchi-Berthouze and A. Kleinsmith, "A categorical approach to affective gesture recognition," *Connection Science,* vol. 15, pp. 259–269, 2003.

[57] J. Sanghvi, G. Castellano, I. Leite, A. Pereira, P. W. McOwan, and A. Paiva, "Automatic analysis of affective postures and body motion to detect engagement with a game companion," in *2011 6th ACM/IEEE international conference on human-robot interaction (HRI),* 2011, pp. 305–311.

[58] K. Vermun, M. Senapaty, A. Sankhla, P. Patnaik, and A. Routray, "Gesture-based affective and cognitive states recognition using kinect for effective feedback during e-learning," in *2013 IEEE fifth international conference on technology for education (T4E)*, 2013, pp. 107–110.

[59] A. Kleinsmith, N. Bianchi-Berthouze, and A. Steed, "Automatic recognition of non-acted affective postures," *IEEE Transactions on Systems, Man, and Cybernetics, Part B (Cybernetics)*, vol. 41, pp. 1027–1038, 2011.

[60] A. Kapur, A. Kapur, N. Virji-Babul, G. Tzanetakis, and P. F. Driessen, "Gesture-based affective computing on motion capture data," in *International conference on affective computing and intelligent interaction*, 2005, pp. 1–7.

[61] D. Bernhardt and P. Robinson, "Detecting affect from non-stylised body motions," in *International conference on affective computing and intelligent interaction*, 2007, pp. 59–70.

[62] D. Bernhardt and P. Robinson, "Detecting emotions from connected action sequences," in *International visual informatics conference*, 2009, pp. 1–11.

[63] M. Karg, K. Kuhnlenz, and M. Buss, "Recognition of affect based on gait patterns," *IEEE Transactions on Systems, Man, and Cybernetics, Part B (Cybernetics)*, vol. 40, pp. 1050–1061, 2010.

[64] N. Savva, A. Scarinzi, and N. Bianchi-Berthouze, "Continuous recognition of player's affective body expression as dynamic quality of aesthetic experience," *IEEE Transactions on Computational Intelligence and AI in games*, vol. 4, pp. 199–212, 2012.

[65] M. Benzeghiba, R. De Mori, O. Deroo, S. Dupont, T. Erbes, D. Jouvet, *et al.*, "Automatic speech recognition and speech variability: A review," *Speech Communication*, vol. 49, pp. 763–786, 2007.

[66] Y. Xia, E. Cambria, A. Hussain, and H. Zhao, "Word polarity disambiguation using bayesian model and opinion-level features," *Cognitive Computation*, vol. 7, pp. 369–380, 2015.

[67] J. M. Chenlo and D. E. Losada, "An empirical study of sentence features for subjectivity and polarity classification," *Information Sciences*, vol. 280, pp. 275–288, 2014.

[68] F. Weninger, M. Wöllmer, and B. Schuller, "Emotion recognition in naturalistic speech and language—a survey," in *Emotion Recognition: A Pattern Analysis Approach*, Hoboken, NJ: John Wiley & Sons, Inc., 2015, pp. 237–267.

[69] B. Schuller, A. Batliner, D. Seppi, S. Steidl, T. Vogt, J. Wagner, et al., "The relevance of feature type for the automatic classification of emotional user states: low level descriptors and functionals," in *Proc. INTERSPEECH*, Antwerp, Belgium, 2007, pp. 2253–2256.

[70] R. Banse and K. R. Scherer, "Acoustic profiles in vocal emotion expression," *Journal of Personality and Social Psychology*, vol. 70, p. 614, 1996.

[71] C. Jones and J. Sutherland, "Acoustic emotion recognition for affective computer gaming," in *Affect and emotion in human-computer interaction*, Berlin Heidelberg, Germany: Springer, 2008, pp. 209–219.

[72] F. Eyben, M. Wöllmer, and B. Schuller, "OpenEAR—introducing the Munich open-source emotion and affect recognition toolkit," in *2009 3rd international conference on affective computing and intelligent interaction and workshops*, 2009, pp. 1–6.

[73] S. Wu, T. H. Falk, and W.-Y. Chan, "Automatic speech emotion recognition using modulation spectral features," *Speech Communication*, vol. 53, pp. 768–785, 2011.

[74] B. Schuller, R. Müller, F. Eyben, J. Gast, B. Hörnler, M. Wöllmer, *et al.*, "Being bored? Recognising natural interest by extensive audiovisual integration for real-life application," *Image and Vision Computing*, vol. 27, pp. 1760–1774, 2009.

[75] B. Schuller and G. Rigoll, "Recognising interest in conversational speech-comparing bag of frames and supra-segmental features," in *Proc. INTERSPEECH*, Brighton, UK, 2009, pp. 1999–2002.

[76] T. Vogt, E. André, and J. Wagner, "Automatic recognition of emotions from speech: A review of the literature and recommendations for practical realisation," in *Affect and emotion in human-computer interaction*, Berlin Heidelberg, Germany: Springer, 2008, pp. 75–91.

[77] A. Stuhlsatz, C. Meyer, F. Eyben, T. Zielke, G. Meier, and B. Schuller, "Deep neural networks for acoustic emotion recognition: Raising the benchmarks," in *2011 IEEE international conference on acoustics, speech and signal processing (ICASSP)*, 2011, pp. 5688–5691.

[78] J. Deng, Z. Zhang, E. Marchi, and B. Schuller, "Sparse autoencoder-based feature transfer learning for speech emotion recognition," in *2013 Humaine Association Conference on Affective Computing and Intelligent Interaction (ACII)*, 2013, pp. 511–516.

[79] L. Li, Y. Zhao, D. Jiang, Y. Zhang, F. Wang, I. Gonzalez, *et al.*, "Hybrid deep neural network-Hidden Markov Model (DNN-HMM) based speech emotion recognition," in *2013 humaine association conference on affective computing and intelligent interaction (ACII)*, 2013, pp. 312–317.

[80] T. Dalgleish, B. D. Dunn, and D. Mobbs, "Affective neuroscience: Past, present, and future," *Emotion Review*, vol. 1, pp. 355–368, 2009.

[81] M.-Z. Poh, D. J. McDuff, and R. W. Picard, "Advancements in noncontact, multiparameter physiological measurements using a webcam," *IEEE Transactions on Biomedical Engineering*, vol. 58, pp. 7–11, 2011.

[82] D. McDuff, S. Gontarek, and R. W. Picard, "Improvements in remote cardiopulmonary measurement using a five band digital camera," *IEEE Transactions on Biomedical Engineering*, vol. 61, pp. 2593–2601, 2014.

[83] J. A. Healey and R. W. Picard, "Detecting stress during real-world driving tasks using physiological sensors," *IEEE Transactions on Intelligent Transportation Systems*, vol. 6, pp. 156–166, 2005.

[84] N. Hjortskov, D. Rissén, A. K. Blangsted, N. Fallentin, U. Lundberg, and K. Søgaard, "The effect of mental stress on heart rate variability and blood pressure during computer work," *European Journal of Applied Physiology*, vol. 92, pp. 84–89, 2004.

[85] E. Jovanov, A. D. Lords, D. Raskovic, P. G. Cox, R. Adhami, and F. Andrasik, "Stress monitoring using a distributed wireless intelligent sensor system," *IEEE Engineering in Medicine and Biology Magazine,* vol. 22, pp. 49–55, 2003.

[86] A. Nakasone, H. Prendinger, and M. Ishizuka, "Emotion recognition from electromyography and skin conductance," in *Proc. of the 5th international workshop on biosignal interpretation,* 2005, pp. 219–222.

[87] G. Chanel, J. Kronegg, D. Grandjean, and T. Pun, "Emotion assessment: Arousal evaluation using EEG's and peripheral physiological signals," in *International workshop on multimedia content representation, classification and security,* 2006, pp. 530–537.

[88] Z. Khalili and M. Moradi, "Emotion detection using brain and peripheral signals," in *2008 Cairo international biomedical engineering conference,* 2008, pp. 1–4.

[89] R. Horlings, D. Datcu, and L. J. Rothkrantz, "Emotion recognition using brain activity," in *Proceedings of the 9th international conference on computer systems and technologies and workshop for PhD students in computing,* 2008, p. 6.

[90] R. Gupta and T. H. Falk, "Relevance vector classifier decision fusion and EEG graph-theoretic features for automatic affective state characterization," *Neurocomputing,* vol. 174, pp. 875–884, 2016.

[91] A. Clerico, R. Gupta, and T. H. Falk, "Mutual information between inter-hemispheric EEG spectro-temporal patterns: A new feature for automated affect recognition," in *2015 7th international IEEE/EMBS conference on neural engineering (NER),* 2015, pp. 914–917.

[92] I. Homma and Y. Masaoka, "Breathing rhythms and emotions," *Experimental Physiology,* vol. 93, pp. 1011–1021, 2008.

[93] S. E. Rimm-Kaufman and J. Kagan, "The psychological significance of changes in skin temperature," *Motivation and Emotion,* vol. 20, pp. 63–78, 1996.

[94] G. Hughes, "On the mean accuracy of statistical pattern recognizers," *IEEE Transactions on Information Theory,* vol. 14, pp. 55–63, 1968.

[95] F. Lingenfelser, J. Wagner, and E. André, "A systematic discussion of fusion techniques for multi-modal affect recognition tasks," in *Proceedings of the 13th international conference on multimodal interfaces,* 2011, pp. 19–26.

[96] J. Wagner, E. Andre, F. Lingenfelser, and J. Kim, "Exploring fusion methods for multimodal emotion recognition with missing data," *IEEE Transactions on Affective Computing,* vol. 2, pp. 206–218, 2011.

[97] L. A. Alexandre, A. C. Campilho, and M. Kamel, "On combining classifiers using sum and product rules," *Pattern Recognition Letters,* vol. 22, pp. 1283–1289, 2001.

[98] C. Y. Suen and L. Lam, "Multiple classifier combination methodologies for different output levels," in *International workshop on multiple classifier systems,* 2000, pp. 52–66.

[99] L. Lam and C. Y. Suen, "Optimal combinations of pattern classifiers," *Pattern Recognition Letters,* vol. 16, pp. 945–954, 1995.

[100] Y. S. Huang and C. Y. Suen, "The behavior-knowledge space method for combination of multiple classifiers," in *IEEE computer society conference on computer vision and pattern recognition*, 1993, pp. 347–347.

[101] R. Gupta, M. Khomami Abadi, J. A. Cárdenes Cabré, F. Morreale, T. H. Falk, and N. Sebs, "A quality adaptive multimodal affect recognition system for user-centric multimedia indexing," in *Proceedings of the 2016 ACM on international conference on multimedia retrieval*, 2016, pp. 317–320.

[102] J. Kim and F. Lingenfelser, "Ensemble approaches to parametric decision fusion for bimodal emotion recognition," in *Proc. BIOSIGNALS*, Valencia, Spain, 2010, pp. 460–463.

[103] M. E. Tipping, "Sparse Bayesian learning and the relevance vector machine," *Journal of Machine Learning Research*, vol. 1, pp. 211–244, 2001.

[104] J. Kim, E. André, M. Rehm, T. Vogt, and J. Wagner, "Integrating information from speech and physiological signals to achieve emotional sensitivity," in *Proc. INTERSPEECH*, Lisboa, Portugal, 2005, pp. 809–812.

[105] M. F. Valstar and M. Pantic, "Combined support vector machines and hidden markov models for modeling facial action temporal dynamics," in *International workshop on human-computer interaction*, 2007, pp. 118–127.

[106] F. Ringeval, B. Schuller, M. Valstar, S. Jaiswal, E. Marchi, D. Lalanne, *et al.*, "Av+ ec 2015: The first affect recognition challenge bridging across audio, video, and physiological data," in *Proceedings of the 5th international workshop on audio/visual emotion challenge*, 2015, pp. 3–8.

[107] S. Jerritta, M. Murugappan, R. Nagarajan, and K. Wan, "Physiological signals based human emotion recognition: a review," in *2011 IEEE 7th international colloquium on signal processing and its applications (CSPA)*, 2011, pp. 410–415.

[108] O. Martin, I. Kotsia, B. Macq, and I. Pitas, "The eNTERFACE'05 audio-visual emotion database," in *22nd international conference on data engineering workshops (ICDEW'06)*, 2006, pp. 8–8.

[109] A. Dhall, R. Goecke, S. Lucey, T. Gedeon, "Collecting large, richly annotated facial-expression databases from movies," *IEEE Multimedia*, vol. 19, pp. 34–31, 2012.

[110] J. D. Morris, "Observations: SAM: the Self-Assessment Manikin; an efficient cross-cultural measurement of emotional response," *Journal of Advertising Research*, vol. 35, pp. 63–68, 1995.

[111] R. Cowie, E. Douglas-Cowie, S. Savvidou*, E. McMahon, M. Sawey, and M. Schröder, "'FEELTRACE': An instrument for recording perceived emotion in real time," in *ISCA tutorial and research workshop (ITRW) on speech and emotion*, 2000.

[112] T. Bänziger, M. Mortillaro, and K. R. Scherer, "Introducing the Geneva multimodal expression corpus for experimental research on emotion perception," *Emotion*, vol. 12, p. 1161, 2012.

[113] E. Douglas-Cowie, R. Cowie, C. Cox, N. Amier, and D. Heylen, "The sensitive artificial listner: An induction technique for generating emotionally coloured conversation," 2008.

[114] E. Douglas-Cowie, R. Cowie, and M. Schröder, "A new emotion database: Considerations, sources and scope," in *ISCA tutorial and research workshop (ITRW) on speech and emotion*, 2000.

[115] E. Douglas-Cowie, R. Cowie, I. Sneddon, C. Cox, O. Lowry, M. Mcrorie, *et al.*, "The HUMAINE database: addressing the collection and annotation of naturalistic and induced emotional data," in *International conference on affective computing and intelligent interaction*, 2007, pp. 488–500.

[116] M. Grimm, K. Kroschel, and S. Narayanan, "The Vera am Mittag German audio-visual emotional speech database," in *2008 IEEE international conference on multimedia and expo*, 2008, pp. 865–868.

[117] G. McKeown, M. F. Valstar, R. Cowie, and M. Pantic, "The SEMAINE corpus of emotionally coloured character interactions," in *2010 IEEE international conference on multimedia and expo (ICME)*, 2010, pp. 1079–1084.

[118] S. Koelstra, C. Muhl, M. Soleymani, J.-S. Lee, A. Yazdani, T. Ebrahimi, *et al.*, "Deap: A database for emotion analysis; using physiological signals," *IEEE Transactions on Affective Computing*, vol. 3, pp. 18–31, 2012.

[119] F. Ringeval, A. Sonderegger, J. Sauer, and D. Lalanne, "Introducing the RECOLA multimodal corpus of remote collaborative and affective interactions," in *2013 10th IEEE international conference and workshops on automatic face and gesture recognition (FG)*, 2013, pp. 1–8.

[120] R. Gupta, H. J. Banville, and T. H. Falk, "PhySyQX: A database for physiological evaluation of synthesised speech quality-of-experience," in *2015 IEEE workshop on applications of signal processing to audio and acoustics (WASPAA)*, 2015, pp. 1–5.

[121] H. Kaya and A. A. Salah, "Combining modality-specific extreme learning machines for emotion recognition in the wild," in *Proceedings of the 16th international conference on multimodal interaction*, 2014, pp. 487–493.

[122] P. Rani, C. Liu, N. Sarkar, and E. Vanman, "An empirical study of machine learning techniques for affect recognition in human–robot interaction," *Pattern Analysis and Applications*, vol. 9, pp. 58–69, 2006.

[123] A. Kapoor, W. Burleson, and R. W. Picard, "Automatic prediction of frustration," *International journal of human-computer studies*, vol. 65, pp. 724–736, 2007.

[124] S. K. D'mello and J. Kory, "A review and meta-analysis of multimodal affect detection systems," *ACM Computing Surveys (CSUR)*, vol. 47, p. 43, 2015.

[125] C. E. Izard, "Innate and universal facial expressions: evidence from developmental and cross-cultural research," 1994.

[126] U. Hess, R. Banse, and A. Kappas, "The intensity of facial expression is determined by underlying affective state and social situation," *Journal of personality and social psychology*, vol. 69, p. 280, 1995.

[127] Z. Zeng, M. Pantic, G. I. Roisman, and T. S. Huang, "A survey of affect recognition methods: Audio, visual, and spontaneous expressions," *IEEE transactions on pattern analysis and machine intelligence*, vol. 31, pp. 39–58, 2009.

[128] J. Kim, "Bimodal emotion recognition using speech and physiological changes", *Robust Speech Recognition and Understanding*, pp. 265–280, 2007.

[129] K. Forbes-Riley and D. J. Litman, "Predicting emotion in spoken dialogue from multiple knowledge sources," in *HLT-NAACL*, 2004, pp. 201–208.

[130] D. J. Litman and K. Forbes-Riley, "Predicting student emotions in computer-human tutoring dialogues," in *Proceedings of the 42nd annual meeting on association for computational linguistics*, 2004, p. 351.

[131] A. Metallinou, M. Wollmer, A. Katsamanis, F. Eyben, B. Schuller, and S. Narayanan, "Context-sensitive learning for enhanced audiovisual emotion classification," *IEEE Transactions on Affective Computing*, vol. 3, pp. 184–198, 2012.

[132] R. Gupta, S. Arndt, J.-N. Antons, S. Möllery, and T. H. Falk, "Characterization of human emotions and preferences for text-to-speech systems using multimodal neuroimaging methods," in *2014 IEEE 27th Canadian conference on electrical and computer engineering (CCECE)*, 2014, pp. 1–5.